YOU ARE
WHAT YOU EAT

YOU ARE
WHAT YOU EAT

A COMMON-SENSE GUIDE TO
THE MODERN AMERICAN DIET

SARA GILBERT

MACMILLAN PUBLISHING CO., INC.
NEW YORK

Macmillan Publishing Co., Inc.
866 Third Avenue, New York, N.Y. 10022
Collier Macmillan Canada, Ltd.

Printed in the United States of America

10   9   8   7   6   5   4   3   2   1

LIBRARY OF CONGRESS CATALOGING IN PUBLICATION DATA

Gilbert, Sara D   You are what you eat.

Bibliography: p.   Includes index.
SUMMARY: Examines the American diet and offers
teenagers advice on eating nutritiously. Also dis-
cusses the reliability of government protection and
the world food crisis.
1. Nutrition—Juvenile literature.   2. Diet—

ISBN 0-02-736020-2

For Dee, who knew about books and about food.

ACKNOWLEDGMENTS

I started this book with an open mind and with little background other than my experience as a concerned eater, shopper and cook. I am grateful to a number of individuals and organizations for filling in the gaps in my knowledge.

Special thanks go to Ruth Lowenberg, M.S., R.D., Nutritionist, Cooperative Extension Service, New York State Department of Agriculture, for reading the manuscript and offering suggestions and guidance.

For their generosity in contributing their time and ideas during personal interviews, I would like to thank Dr. Joan Gussow, Program Coordinator of the Nutrition Department, Teachers College (Columbia University); Judith Hirshon, head nutritionist with the Children and Youth Program, Roosevelt Hospital (New York); Frank McLaughlin and Howard Seltzer of the U.S. Office of Consumer Affairs; Dr. Kristen McNutt of the Nutrition Foundation,

Inc.; Eleanor Martin and Helen Conway of the Bureau of Nutrition, New York City Health Department; Dr. Lester Tepley and Bjorn Berndtson of UNICEF; the Upper School class members of the Town School, New York City; and Robert Wersan of the Protein-Calorie Advisory Group of the United Nations.

I would like to express my gratitude to the following people for personally sharing their expertise through correspondence or telephone conversation: Dana Dalrymple, agricultural economist with the U.S. Department of Agriculture and the U.S. Agency for International Development; Corelli David, dietician (retired) from the Montgomery County, Maryland, school system; Ruth Desmond, of the Federation of Homemakers, Inc.; Jean Farmer; Lenora Moragne, Director of Nutrition, Child Feeding Program, U.S. Department of Agriculture; and Dr. Frederick Stare, Chairman, Department of Nutrition, Harvard University School of Public Health.

These organizations, agencies and companies have kindly contributed information and material: Action for Children's Television; Agri-business Accountability Project; American Cancer Society; American Dietetic Association; American Farm Bureau Federation; American Home Economics Association; American Institute of Nutrition; American Meat Institute; American Medical Association, Committee on Foods and Nutrition; Center for Disease Control, U.S. Department of Health, Education and Welfare; Center for Science in the Public Interest; Children's Bureau, U.S. Department of Health, Education and Welfare; Consumers' Federation of America; Dairy Council of Metropolitan New York; FMC Corporation; Foremost-McKesson, Inc.; National Dairy Council; National Farmers Union; National Livestock and Meat Board; *Progressive Grocer* magazine; U.S. Department of Agriculture, Agricultural Research Service and Department of Foods and Nutrition; U.S. Senate, Select Committee on Nutrition and Human Needs (George McGovern, Chairman).

CONTENTS

YOU ARE
WHAT YOU EAT

ONE
YOU ARE WHAT YOU EAT

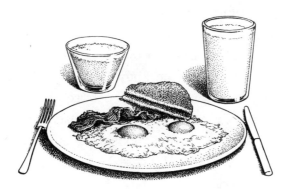

What did you eat for breakfast this morning? A bowl of cereal? A glass of instant breakfast drink? Bacon and eggs? Granola, figs and goat's milk? What difference does it make anyway? If you're like most people you just don't think about it.

Thinking about food is something few Americans do. You may even have had a hard time remembering what you ate for breakfast. You have your likes and dislikes, of course. You may have some definite food habits, such as eating the same kind of breakfast today as you did yesterday and the day before. But beyond that, you probably don't think much about food. You take it for granted.

You take the safety, purity and freshness of your food for granted because you have come to rely on the government to protect you. But the quality of that protection is being questioned now that the food industry, and life itself, have grown so complicated.

You take it for granted that you're eating a good diet. You may think you know what's good for you, but you really *don't*. Your school requires algebra, physics and French, but it doesn't teach you much about food. Most of what you learn about "nutrition" comes from the back of a cereal box or an ad on TV.

Most Americans take food for granted because they can afford to. Our land is and always has been so abundant that few of us, and relatively few of our ancestors, have ever known real starvation. Most of us can always eat something for breakfast.

But you really *can't* afford to take food for granted. The facts are that:

. . . what you eat makes a difference in how you look, how you feel, how well you do in school and how much energy you have.

. . . Americans are getting poorer nutrition than they used to;

. . . teen-agers, people ten to sixteen years old, are the most poorly nourished of any age group in this country;

. . . during adolescence, perhaps more than at any other time in your life, it is essential that you eat the right amounts of the right kinds of foods. You are growing faster now than you have since you were a baby and you need proper nutrition for all that growth, change and activity—what you eat or don't eat now can affect you for the rest of your life.

Food is vital to life. It is also central to all of the major social functions in the world. Think about breakfast cereal, for example. The money your family spends for a box of "Flakies" helps bring income to grocery store employees, warehouse workers, truckers, processors, farmers and all the other people and businesses that depend on them. That's *economics.*

On the other hand, in 1975 the farmer got three dollars a bushel for grain that cost the consumer seventy-five dollars a bushel when it was packaged and sold in the store. The way in which farmers, food industry executives, government officials and our elected representatives try to regulate the price of grain is called *politics.*

If the grain that went into Flakies were available, unprocessed, to a hungry family, it might hold off starvation. Who should get the grain, you or they? When we deal with issues like this, we're talking about philosophy and *morality.*

According to some estimates, over a billion people

suffer from severe hunger or malnutrition, at least during part of the year. The way in which the United States hands out or holds on to its food supply is a matter of *diplomacy,* and it could make the difference between war and peace in your lifetime.

Nutrition, politics, economics, morality, diplomacy—these are not the kinds of things you usually think about over your breakfast cereal. But they are ideas you need to deal with. These fancy words and faraway problems are going to have a personal impact on you.

TWO
PASS YOUR PLATE

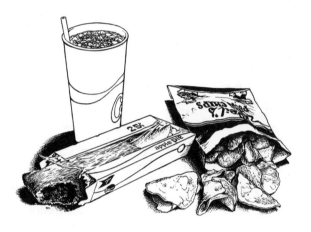

If you are like most teen-agers, you probably skip or skimp on breakfast. You may not eat much for lunch, either, especially if that meal is of the all-too-common lunchroom variety. You make up for those missing calories by snacking a lot—a candy bar or soda between classes, a pizza or hamburger after school, potato chips and soda while studying or watching TV.

If you are weight-conscious, you may try to avoid foods you consider "high-calorie," such as milk or breads and other "starches." If you are athletic, you probably go in for foods you consider "body-building proteins," like milk and meat. No matter who you are, it's a good bet that you shy away from most vegetables and dig into any food that's sweet.

The above is only a general picture, based on nutritional studies and observations of typical teen-age diets. It may not describe your particular pattern.

THE AMERICAN WAY

Individual food habits vary by region, by ethnic background, by family styles and income and by individual tastes. However, it is possible to make some general comments on the American diet.

VARIETY: Foreigners are amazed (and our own great-grandparents would be too) at the different types of foods available to most Americans. A good-sized supermarket is stocked with over ten thousand separate items, and the number keeps increasing. Variety throughout the year and across the country is possible because of American technology. The food industry can preserve almost any kind of food by canning, concentrating, freezing, drying, freeze-drying or by adding a chemical preservative. Variety is important because it's enjoyable and because it tends to insure the nutritional balance the body requires.

Food can travel so swiftly that it's possible, if costly, for a family in the northeast to eat Hawaiian pineapples, California lettuce or Texas watermelons during the long, cold winter. You eat South American bananas, New Zealand lamb or African grapes without thinking about the journey that the food must take to reach your table.

SAFETY: We're safer than most. The food we eat is generally free from the organisms that bring salmonellosis, botulism, typhoid, cholera and other food-borne diseases to people whose countries lack the sanitary facilities and governmental standards that guard our food supply. Whether our food is safe from other dangerous ingredients is another question.

PLENTY: Most Americans have more than enough to eat. The average American takes in about 3100 calories each day—more than the average citizen of most other countries. We eat more proteins and fats, and relatively fewer carbohydrates than most other nationalities. Altogether, we have available more than we need for healthy survival. And there's more where that came from. American agriculture is the most productive in the world, and even when food is scarce elsewhere, we usually have extra.

THE HUNGRY DON'T DIE: Of course, not all Americans

are well fed. Millions of people in our country do not have enough to eat, because they haven't the money to spend on "variety" and "plenty." They endure the pain of hunger and they suffer some of the effects of malnutrition. But few of our citizens actually die from starvation. With help from welfare payments, food stamps and school feeding programs, even the poor manage to eat enough to survive.

OUR HABITS ARE CHANGING: American eating habits have changed a lot during this century, and the rate of change has accelerated over the last few decades. We drink less milk than previously. We don't eat as many fresh fruits and vegetables as we used to. You eat more poultry and beef than your parents did when they were your age, and probably less pork and lamb. Each of us, whether we realize it or not, consumes more grain than Americans did in the past (though we eat much of it indirectly as baked goods, packaged cereals and meat from grain-fed animals). Our tastes are becoming standardized too. Research indicates that ethnic and regional food patterns are blending into more of an "all-American" diet than was once the case.

WE EAT OUT MORE: In 1975, thirty-five cents of every food dollar was spent on food eaten away from home, as compared with just a few pennies in 1950. It's estimated that by 1980 we'll be spending half of our food money eating out. On an average, at least one person in every family eats at least one meal a day in some kind of restaurant or snack shop or in a cafeteria at a school, factory or other institution. You may take these meals away from home for granted, but to your grandparents' generation or to someone from anywhere else in the world, they would be unusual.

WE EAT ON THE RUN: Whether we eat out or at home, we tend not to sit down together for our meals. You may eat toast at the kitchen counter or munch a hot dog on the way to the movies. Your mother may lunch on an apple at the grocery store and your father may have a sandwich supper in front of the TV.

WE SNACK A LOT: Much of our food eaten on the run is snack food. Each year we eat billions of dollars worth of snacks—foods we don't need for health. In 1975, Americans spent $1.5 billion on potato chips, and $50 million on Twinkies snack cakes alone. The food industry counts on selling us more snack foods each year. Even families with only a little money for food spend a lot of it on all the munchies, sweets and fizzies that are a part of our everyday lives.

WE LOOK FOR CONVENIENCE: More than half of the foods most Americans eat are processed foods, and by 1980 that proportion will reach two-thirds. "Processing" includes canning and freezing, of course, but an increasing number of those processed items are classed as "convenience foods"—snacks, frozen dinners or mixes. These products have been partially or completely prepared before marketing, so that little or none of the cooking is done in the home. We pay for the processing that makes this convenience possible, but many Americans seem to feel that freedom from the kitchen is worth the price.

IT COSTS MORE: In general, Americans pay more each year for food than they did the year before. As inflation continues and resources grow scarce, costs go up. Your family may also be spending a larger proportion of its income on food than it used to. Economists have usually estimated that Americans spend an average of 17 percent of their financial resources for food, though of course that percentage increases as an individual family's income decreases. And now the averages are rising, too. Processed foods, food shipped long distances and restaurant meals cost more than foods grown near home and cooked in the kitchen.

IT COMES IN BULK: Until fairly recently, most

Americans shopped at small, locally owned stores whose shelves were stocked with food raised or packaged by nearby farmers or factories. Today we buy most of our food from supermarkets owned by a rather small number of regional or national chains. Their stock comes from a relatively few huge processing companies, which in turn purchase supplies from a dwindling number of increasingly large farms. The food industry boasts that the advantages of such concentration of food power are efficiency and lowered unit cost. But there are disadvantages, too, as will be noted later.

WE'RE MORE CONCERNED: The late 1960s saw the beginning of increased interest in good nutrition and concern over food quality, and food awareness has been growing ever since. We are beginning to think about what we eat and about what we're missing. And that's a good thing, for there is cause for concern. Despite all the advantages our diet offers, there are also many disadvantages. What you don't know about food *can* hurt you.

THREE
EAT!

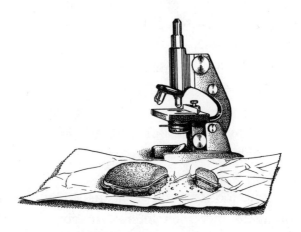

Your body is a self-contained system; it is constantly creating, defending and re-creating itself. It operates automatically, so that you are not aware of what's happening inside you unless some part of the system breaks down.

The things your body needs for life and growth are simple to list: proteins, fats, carbohydrates, vitamins, minerals, water and oxygen, plus some fiber. What your body does with those nutrients is not so simple; in fact, it's quite complex.

Your body is like a sophisticated chemical laboratory run by a computer (your brain). It takes in the raw materials, breaks them down through the process of digestion into their simplest forms and converts them into new forms by a process called metabolism.

The products of digestion are sent, via the bloodstream, throughout the system. Each of the body's billions of cells is programmed to take from the blood exactly the ingredients it needs to perform its specific functions.

Protein, in the form of amino acids, goes to build and repair all tissues, to produce enzymes and hormones, which regulate the body's processes, and to make antibodies, which protect the body from disease.

Fats, as fatty acids, aid digestion and carry vitamins. Fats are stored for future energy needs and as padding to protect nerves and organs.

Carbohydrates, as simple sugars, are the main source of the energy that fuels all the body's external activities as well as its internal functions, including thought.

Minerals strengthen the cells of bones, blood and organs. Vitamins help regulate the body's functions and combine with other nutrients to maintain health. Fiber helps keep the digestive system moving by forcing food through and out of the digestive tract.

Water carries all these raw materials, removes wastes, maintains body temperature and provides the fluid in which the cells carry out all the complex chemical changes that make for life. Oxygen combines with other nutrients to make these transformations possible.

It is hard for most of us to think of a ham sandwich in terms of biochemistry. But in a very real sense you *are* what you eat, and if you want to look good, feel good, think clearly and be able to enjoy life, you've got to provide your body with the right kind of food in the right amounts and in the right proportions.

The energy value of food is expressed in calories. A calorie is simply a unit for the measurement of energy, as an inch or a centimeter is a unit for the measurement of length. The calories you take in need to be divided proportionately among proteins, fats and carbohydrates. The proportions are important because each ingredient helps make the others effective. For example, if you don't get enough carbohydrate, you can't make proper use of the fats in your diet; without adequate fat intake, you can't make use of vitamins A, D, E or K, no matter what quantity of vitamins you take in.

In the back of this book is a chart that lists the number of calories and the proportions of nutrients for a person your age. It explains what they're for and suggests sources for obtaining them. Compare your eating habits against the chart to see if you are getting what you need. You may be surprised at what you're missing or getting too much of.

WE ARE ALL EXPERTS

Few of us have any clear idea of what we really eat, let alone what we need. But most of us *think* we know what's good for us. We consider ourselves experts about our own food, so we latch on to each nutrition fad that hits the headlines and we gobble up each new taste treat.

To be a real expert in nutrition is hard. For one thing, many people think nutrition is boring. It's also a highly complex subject, and an expert in, say, its biochemical aspects may be ignorant of dietetics. As the conflicting results of some nutrition surveys indicate, even the experts have a hard time agreeing. For example, one government study indicates that many teen-aged boys get too little calcium and iron, but another study shows that they eat enough of everything except vitamin C. A nationwide survey lists the diets of teen-aged girls as low in many nutrients; other research shows that they do not get enough of *anything* (including protein) except for two B vitamins and vitamin A. Whom should you believe? It's confusing.

Few people will take the time and trouble to understand such a complicated topic, no matter how important it is. Few schools teach nutrition well; those that do teach it are often out of date.

MISSING INGREDIENTS

Given the abundance and variety of the American diet, each of us should be able to get all of the nutrients we need without even thinking about it. But we don't.

Of the various recent nutrition surveys, the most thorough was conducted by the federal government in 1965. It found that, in general, Americans suffered serious deficiencies of calcium and iron and tended to short themselves on vitamins A and C. It showed that one-fifth of the population ate "poorly," that is, consumed less than two-thirds of the Recommended Daily Allowances of the nutrients officially classified as essential. Compared with a similar study made in 1955, the survey indicated that more Americans were eating fewer of the essentials.

When we eat poorly, we suffer for it. Our bones and teeth can weaken and become brittle with age from lack of calcium. Insufficient vitamin A and vitamin C can make us vulnerable to frequent colds, slow-healing wounds and bruises, skin and mucous irritations, gum diseases and poor vision. Without enough of the B vitamins, our digestion is poor and we tend to be nervous, depressed and apathetic.

Recent preliminary research shows that Americans may also take in too little fiber. Fiber—roughage or "bulk"—is the part of food that the body cannot digest (the hulls of whole grains, for instance). Fiber passes through the digestive system almost intact and acts like a plumber's snake to keep the tract cleared out. Some doctors think that without enough fiber, our digestion may become too slow, leaving us susceptible to intestinal diseases, including, perhaps, cancer. On the other hand, too much fiber or a sudden increase in fiber intake can also interfere with digestion.

Other tentative studies have linked nutritional deficiencies to various forms of mental illness. It has been shown that without adequate nutrition, the body and the mind lack the strength to withstand physical and emotional stress. People can be tired, nervous and irritable; they can have poor skin, indigestion or bad teeth and it *might* all be due to something they didn't eat.

TOO LITTLE

The deficiency diseases most of us may live with are mild compared with those that some people suffer:

KWASHIORKOR AND MARASMUS: two exotic names

for the same problem—starvation. Countless people in the world, most of them children, are dwarfed, twisted or brain-damaged because of a serious, continuing lack of calories, protein or both.

BERIBERI: weakness in all the muscles, including the heart, due to inadequate thiamin (a B vitamin).

RICKETS: soft and twisted bones as a result of too little vitamin D.

SCURVY: pain, swelling and excessive bleeding due to insufficient vitamin C.

XEROPHTHALMIA: eye irritation and blindness from too little vitamin A.

ARIBOFLAVINOSIS: blurred vision and skin sores due to insufficient riboflavin (a B vitamin).

PELLAGRA: listlessness and poor digestion as a result of too little niacin (another B vitamin).

GOITER: swollen thyroid gland, a symptom of insufficient iodine (a mineral found in sea water, iodized salt and some soils).

Not all nutritional diseases have such fancy names, but they are no less serious. Poor nutrition can lead to birth defects. And, if a baby is not properly nourished while it is growing in its mother's womb, it will not be healthy when born. This cycle of malnutrition—weak babies from poorly fed mothers—is a major problem among poverty-stricken families everywhere in the world. A teen-aged girl who becomes pregnant has a doubly difficult task: feeding herself adequately for her own growth and nourishing the baby that is growing within her.

Inadequate food early in life can cause brain damage and mental retardation. It's sometimes hard to realize that our brains are a part of our bodies. Since we think with them, we tend to imagine them as somehow detached from the rest of us. But they're not. Like the rest of our bodies, our brains are composed of cells. The cells are supplied with food by the blood. If the blood has insufficient food the brain cannot grow or function properly.

People who eat poorly may not show the symptoms of any official form of malnutrition, but they may leave their bodies open to attack by the germs of other diseases. You have probably found that when you let yourself get too tired or too "run-down" you are more likely to catch a cold than at other times. People who have had too little to eat for a long time, are vulnerable to diseases worse than colds.

TOO MUCH

Those of us who have enough to eat can suffer from too much of a good thing. Let's look at some of the more immediate effects of an overabundant diet:

OBESITY: a major health problem in the United States. We eat more than we need and we get fat. Overweight is linked to early death from heart disease, diabetes and stroke, and it makes treatment of other ailments difficult. People who carry too much body weight can't move well, which makes it difficult to get enough exercise, and this can throw the entire system out of whack.

"EMPTY CALORIES": foods that provide little or no nutrition. Sweets, sugar and many snack foods provide little but calories. When we fill our stomachs with them, we miss out on the nutrients that other foods offer, and we become fat *and* undernourished.

DENTAL CARIES: cavities, or holes in the teeth. Too much sugar can eat away at the coating of the teeth. Americans ate an average of ninety pounds of sugar per person in 1975, and that adds up to a lot of cavities.

"HARDENING OF THE ARTERIES": a condition resulting from the layering of the blood vessels with plaque —fats and fatlike substances, including cholesterol. People whose diets are built around fat meats and other "rich" foods tend to lay down a coating of fatty and fibrous substances in their blood vessels and they may suffer heart disease and stroke as a result. Men in our society are the most frequent victims, but all young people can start setting themselves up for hardening of the arteries early in life if they're not careful.

CANCER: perhaps the most dread disease of modern times. Cancers of various types have been linked to the overintake of fats and refined foods and the underintake of fiber. Studies show, for example, that rural Africans, whose diet is high in fiber and extremely low in fat, suffer almost no cancer of the colon. Among Africans who live in more "westernized" cities (and whose diet is higher in fat and lower in fiber), the colon-cancer rate is higher; while among American Blacks, this cancer is one of the leading causes of death, as it is for the American population as a whole. Other research indicates that breast cancer may be related to a high fat intake and that other cancers may result from deficiencies in vitamins A and C or from the intake of food additives.

Thus abundance, sugar and rich meats—the hallmarks of "advanced" and wealthy civilizations—are also the causes of our major nutrition-related diseases. We indulge ourselves and end up with cavities, cancer and heart attacks in numbers not suffered by "less privileged" societies.

IS IT SAFE?

As foods become more convenient, they may be growing less safe. Some experts argue that strict sanitation is impossible to maintain given the many stages through which our food passes, leaving us open to food-borne illnesses. A 1975 federal survey found that 90 percent of the nation's restaurants —where we eat so much of our food—may be unsanitary.

But other more serious and widespread diseases can result from food processing. Chemical food technology is such a new field that little is known about any long-term, accumulated effects of many common additives. Some chemicals that are now added to foods to lengthen their "shelf life" or improve their appearance are suspected of contributing to cancer, emotional problems, allergic reactions, birth defects and other disorders.

Some additives, such as lecithin, are useful in keeping food fresh. But many additives serve only to make packaged foods look better or to give the flavor an artificial boost. Many additives offer the consumer no real benefit and many risks. The chart on page 124 lists some common additives, their purposes and their possible dangers.

FOUR

THE TASTE TEST

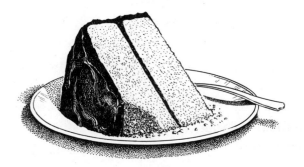

We eat the foods we do because they "taste good." It's as simple as that. But taste is not at all simple.

For one thing, taste is a highly individual matter. "Each to his own taste," we hear, or "One man's meat is another man's poison," and "There's no accounting for taste."

Taste involves personal preferences, cultural influences and emotional needs. Before we get to all that, we need to find out something about taste as a physical sensation.

STICK OUT YOUR TONGUE

Under a microscope, your tongue looks like a hairbrush. The surface is covered with tiny bristles, each of which grows through a pore from a taste bud beneath the tongue's surface. Within each taste bud is a cluster of thin cells which receive flavor information as chewing and saliva spread the food over the tongue. The taste buds pass the information on to the brain.

As you may have noticed when you lick a lollipop with the tip of your tongue or gulp medicine quickly over the back of it, you are sensitive to different flavors in different parts of your mouth. You taste sweetness at the front of the tongue, sourness along the sides, and bitterness at the very back. Taste buds for saltiness are scattered all over the tongue. When you eat a food you really like, you tend to savor it, letting it stay in your mouth for a while. In that way, all the different taste buds are stimulated and the combination gives your brain the pleasant flavor message.

Of course you don't taste only with your taste buds. The sense of smell is an important means of carrying flavor signals, which is why food tastes so "blah" when you have a cold in the nose. Texture and temperature also make a difference in the flavor of a food: the difference between chocolate milk and hot chocolate, for instance, or between scrambled eggs done just right and those that are too soft or too hard.

Just the sight of food can start your mouth watering—and you are ready to begin digesting. Sight can also influence the way food tastes. You probably wouldn't like the taste of green steak or purple French fries.

Your sense of taste is also affected by your age. Your taste buds are probably less sensitive now than they were when you were small. If there's something you hated as a child, try it now—you may not find it so distasteful.

EAT IT AND LIKE IT

If you lived on an island where there was nothing to eat but raw fish, seaweed and coconut milk, you would love raw fish, seaweed and coconut milk. People eat what's available. Not only that, but if they're hungry enough, they'll like whatever they're eating.

If you were born and raised on raw fish and then moved to a place where all you could eat were cheeseburgers, you would have a hard time getting used to them. What you learn to eat early in life, you learn to like, and you tend to keep on eating and enjoying it. You learn your first and strongest food habits from your family. Your family in turn learns them from the society in which it lives.

Whole cultures are built around food and its availability. Oriental societies, for instance, whose food resources have been limited by space and geography, have food rituals that focus on taste from many different angles. A Chinese or Japanese chef can vary the appearance, taste and texture of a few foods so that a small meal gives a lot of eating pleasure.

FOOD FOR THE SOUL

But food is more than simple need or habit. It can be a highly emotional subject, too. To some tribes, certain foods are taboo: it is forbidden to eat them. Probably no member of the tribe could explain *why* a food is taboo, except by quoting an ancient myth —yet no one is allowed to eat it. If all other food gave out, the tribe would probably move or starve rather than eat it.

We also see taboos on a more sophisticated cultural level. To Jewish people who "keep kosher," pork and shellfish are taboo. A kosher Jew may not eat dairy products and meat in one meal, and must use separate plates for the two types of foods.

Until recently Catholics were forbidden meat on Friday and during the weeks preceding Easter. To

Moslems, pork is taboo, as is other meat not properly killed. Pious Hindus are forbidden all meat, many dairy products and even some vegetables.

These taboos originated way back in the histories of these religions. They are so well rooted in the emotional foundations of these faiths that they influence the taste of their followers.

Of course you don't have to be a member of any religion or primitive tribe for food to have emotional and psychological symbolism. We eat with our minds as much as with our tongues, and each of us has many personal associations with various foods. If, as a child, you vomited after eating a large portion of lima beans, you may never like lima beans again. If your mother makes you chicken soup when you're sick, you may always turn to chicken soup when you're feeling down. When a family dinner is accompanied by tension or arguing, the food doesn't taste as good as when everyone is relaxed and happy.

Foods that we associate with comfort or pleasure will always taste better than those that remind us of distress and pain. What are some of your likes and dislikes, and what emotions attach to them?

FOOD AS FUN

A milk shake you sip by yourself doesn't taste quite

as good as the same shake sipped when you're in the company of friends. Eating is the one common denominator we share with everyone else, no matter what our varying interests. Because food brings people together, it is an important part of ceremonies, whether it's the wafer and wine of the Mass, the breaking of the Sabbath loaf or the turkey at Thanksgiving.

We learn to associate certain foods with fun or festivities. If you really concentrate on the flavor of those potato chips, you may decide that the taste is actually not so great. But chips are a "fun food." If your friends considered apples "fun," you would buy apples instead of potato chips.

A food that is "in" tastes better than a food that is "out." Ten years ago, for instance, yogurt was considered "yukky" by most people. Today, it is an "in" food, and the yogurt business is booming.

In a tribe where goat's eyes are reserved for the chief, to be presented with goat's eyes is an honor, and the honor makes them delicious. A woman who barely bothers to boil water for her own family may serve a gourmet feast to guests, not so much because she wants to please them, but because she wants to show how expert or well-off she is. The United Nations Children's Fund (UNICEF) reports that poor villagers, near starvation, will sell their chicken eggs to buy Coca Cola, because Coke carries the status that eggs lack, though it provides no nourishment.

We eat foods, then, because we like them. We like them because they "taste good." We taste, physically, with our tongues, our noses, our eyes, and our brains. But we also *learn* to taste. We like what's available. We enjoy what our culture says is good, and avoid what it says is bad. We like what we are in the habit of eating, whether or not it is good for us. And we taste with our emotions as well; we enjoy foods that are comforting, festive, fun or high in status.

THE AMERICAN SWEET TOOTH

How does sugar taste? It tastes sweet. It stimulates the first group of taste buds on the tongue, and since sugar doesn't need to blend with any other buds to send its flavor message, it is a taste that's easy to identify and learn. Sugar offers little stimulus to the senses of smell or sight, so its odor and appearance are neutral, and it doesn't irritate the other senses in the way some basic flavors can. It dissolves easily on the tongue, giving a quick response.

Sugar is available. Whether you use table sugar or not, you eat sugar every day. You're aware of the sugar in cakes and cookies, candy, soda and desserts. But your kitchen cabinet and refrigerator are filled with foods containing sugar: cereals, packaged mixes of all sorts, ketchup, peanut butter, mayonnaise, canned vegetables, bologna, crackers, bread and baby food. You name it, it probably contains sugar. The label may read "dextrose" or "maltose" or "glucose" or "corn syrup," but it's all sugar.

Mothers' milk is sweet, and sugar is added to infant formulas and baby foods, so sugar is a taste you learn during those crucial early stages of life. Sugar also has emotional overtones. When you were little, your mother gave you a lollipop or a cookie when you were "good"; you got a sweet dessert when you cleaned your plate. When you were being punished, or you were on a diet or had a cavity you had to deny yourself the pleasure of a sweet.

Sugar is associated with ceremonies and fun. The wine of the Jewish sabbath and the Catholic mass is sweet, or is replaced by sugary grape juice. A birthday party would be disappointing without cake, ice cream and candy.

Sugar also carries a high status. If that surprises you, think about it. Refined sugar adds nothing to our diet. It's not a necessity, but a luxury. The more advanced in wealth and status a country is, the more sugar its citizens consume. Sugar was once such a scarcity that sweet pastries and candies were special treats. We still carry that attitude with us.

Sugar has almost no nutritional value, yet each year the average American eats more than ninety pounds of it. If that's not an acquired, socially conditioned taste, nothing is.

LEARNING TO LIKE IT

You have grown up in an age of processed, premixed foods, so when you hear people complaining that things don't taste as good as they used to, you may not share their concern. It's true that some gourmets probably carry the business of taste a bit too far. But things *don't* taste as good as they used to.

What is meant by "good" is a personal view, of course, but have you ever eaten an apple straight off the tree, or a tomato just off the vine? Doesn't that food *really* taste better, smell better and feel juicier than the produce you've bought at the store three weeks after it's been picked? And doesn't a hamburger you've just made really provide more zip and satisfaction than a meal that was born out of a mix.

As we've seen there's more to pleasing your palate than allowing food to pass over your taste buds, and there's a lot more to satisfying your appetite than just filling your stomach.

On the whole, the American taste is tuned to eating soft, bland foods, foods of uniform appearance and consistency. Sounds pretty boring, doesn't it? But we wouldn't continue to eat that way if we didn't like it. How did we learn to like it?

FIVE
UP AGAINST THE PRODUCTION LINE

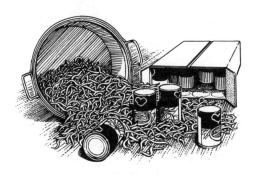

Family style, ethnic background and religious tradition all have some influence on our individual tastes, but to a much larger degree our taste has been shaped by the food business.

The food industry is not in business to develop the subtleties of your palate, to satisfy your moral sensitivity or even to insure your proper nutrition. The food industry is in business to sell food. In the marketplace, food is a product, just as sewing machines, shoes and tractors are products. And like

the makers of those other products, the food manufacturers have found ways to turn out the maximum amount of merchandise for the greatest profit
possible.

Food production is difficult to streamline, because
agriculture—the source of its raw materials—is subject to the whims of nature. But even so, science
and technology have managed to bend nature
enough to make efficiency possible in "agribusiness."

BEANS BY THE BILLION

Let's see how an imaginary food processor manages
to guide its business toward greater profitability
while influencing public food habits and decreasing
the nutritive value of the consumers' diet.

Crunchy Bean Inc., CBI for short, wants to sell
as many cans of beans as possible. That means it
needs a lot of beans to can all year round. It owns,
or has contracts with, hundreds of bean farms
totaling hundreds of thousands of acres in different
parts of the country. The cheapest and quickest way
to harvest all those beans is by machine, so Crunchy
commissions another company to design and build
mechanical bean-pickers. The machines work fine,
but they mangle the beans. The standard farm-
grown green bean, tender enough to eat without
being cooked, is too delicate for machine harvesting.

So CBI scientists develop a seed that produces a strain of bean tough enough to be harvested by machine. The new bean doesn't taste quite as good, but it looks better in the can.

There is an optimum point at which beans should be picked if they are to provide maximum flavor and nutrition. But CBI must transport its beans long distances, and by the time ripe, nourishing beans reach the cannery they're beginning to rot. So the company sees that the beans are harvested before they are at their peak. That way, the beans will be firm at the cannery but not quite so rich in vitamin A.

What does this type of operation mean for the consumer's taste and nutrition? It means that if you ate Crunchy green beans you would be eating food designed for machines, not for people. The beans may not taste as good as those grown on a local farm, but the consumer accepts them because they are more readily available than fresh beans. They have been picked, not at the point at which nature makes them most nutritious, but at the point at which they are the most cannable, but the consumer doesn't know that. They aren't bad for you, but they could be better, and they could taste better.

Of course, our green-bean company is imaginary, but the story is real. And there are countless other examples to choose from.

Tomatoes, for instance, were once a highly perishable and seasonal crop. Now they can be grown and shipped year round. Most "fresh" tomatoes are picked when they're green and reddened artificially with an ethylene gas. They are red and available, but they're hard and tasteless compared with the garden-grown variety, and they lack some of the food value that natural ripening could provide.

To produce meatier animals and speed up growth for increased production, ranchers and poultry farmers add artificial growth hormones to the animal feed. Chickens eat mash containing yellow dye so that their flesh and egg yolks look more "golden." You eventually eat such dyes and growth hormones, and they may not be good for you. Given the opportunity, you could probably taste the difference, too.

There are exceptions to our green-bean model, of course. There are still farmers who raise crops or animals the way they want to, in order to bring about the best-tasting and most nutritionally valuable results possible. They may contract with a few small processors and distributors, or they may be able to afford to get their own crops to market. But to make a profit, they must charge a premium price for their goods because raising high-quality produce in small quantities and selling in small lots costs more per bushel than mass production.

The big money is in mass production and mass

marketing. CBI knows this, and does all it can to increase production and decrease the unit cost.

CREATING A NEED

What happens if people don't want to buy all those cans of beans? CBI loses money. The company has to *make* people want to buy its green beans. If most consumers like green beans soft, not crunchy, CBI will embark on an advertising campaign designed to convince the public that crunchy canned beans are better than "flabby" ones. If the ads work, the public has been "educated" to believe, rightly or wrongly, that canned string beans should be crunchy. Our tastes have altered again.

NEW AND IMPROVED!

If sales pick up, production must be increased. Beans that once could go straight from the trucks into the cans must be kept "fresh" while they wait their turn for processing. To keep them green and firm, CBI sprinkles a preservative over its beans. The preservative isn't harmful, but it adds a certain subtle taste to the beans. And it's not foolproof: while they're sitting, the beans lose a bit more of their nutritive value. Taste changes again, and food value decreases.

Meanwhile, some consumers notice that the beans in the can don't look like the beans on the printed label. The beans in the picture are bright green; the ones in the can are an olive drab. People are complaining. So CBI adds a green dye to its beans, to make them match the label. The customers stop complaining. They have learned that canned beans are supposed to be an emerald green. Any company that tries to sell them beans with the slightly gray tone that naturally results from the canning process is out of luck.

WHAT HAPPENED?

Nature started off with a green bean, a good source of vitamin A and other nutrients. Farmers learned to cultivate that bean, to produce enough to feed a large community during the normal growing season. The beans were flavorful, and rich in nutrition. Commercial canning made it possible for a larger group of people to eat green beans all year round. They tasted all right, and retained much of their original food value.

Then technology and economics stepped in, and, in the end, the vast green-bean public learned to demand canned beans that had been grown tough, picked before they were ripe and artificially preserved and dyed.

What happened to our imaginary bean consumer is what happens to all of us when we buy, taste, eat and learn to like many of the food products on the market today. Most of our food has been grown for appearance and processed for convenience. Taste and nutrition have been left behind.

Of course, the food-processing system is not all bad. Were it not for mass production and the technology of food preservation, we would not have available the wide variety of foods we have today.

But how much *real* variety is there, anyway? Because of the dizzying array of packages that crowd our supermarket shelves, we tend to think that we have a great deal of choice in what we eat. But is it really true?

We may have seven different flavors of corn chips and over a hundred different brands of breakfast cereals, but that kind of "choice" does not represent true variety. If you want to buy five unwaxed apples, you will probably have a hard time—usually you must settle for six waxed ones in a plastic package. If you prefer lamb to beef, you may be out of luck. It's practically impossible to buy cured meats that don't contain nitrites or nitrates. If you decide to avoid dyes and sugar, you will have to give up a large proportion of your standard diet. If you want to buy whole-wheat flour or whole-grain cereals, you have to pay a premium.

The food industry has managed to create thousands of new products and in the process has influenced our tastes and our health. As the number of different food products increases, food quality is decreasing and our actual choice of what to eat is becoming more and more limited.

SIX
BUSINESS IS BOOMING

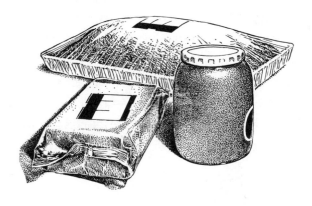

There was a time, not too long ago, when people had little or no choice in their diets. They ate only what they could grow. And if they didn't have a way of storing their harvest from one growing season to the next, they went hungry. If what they could grow lacked essential nutrients, they went without them, living poorly and dying young.

People in some parts of the world live that way today: from hand to mouth, alternating hungry seasons with full ones and never getting quite enough of everything they need. This kind of life allows little time or energy for anything but food—planting it, praying over it, picking it and wondering where the next meal will come from.

Only after people have discovered ways of maintaining a nearly constant food supply, through gardening and domesticating animals, can they afford to develop art, architecture, industry, philosophy and all the other branches of human culture. Since its beginnings some nine thousand years ago, agriculture has made slow but steady progress, with farmers in different areas developing methods suited to getting the most out of their particular land.

LAND OF PLENTY

America is truly the land of plenty. No other part of the world has a better combination of climate, soil and landscape for growing such a wide variety of foods. The early European settlers realized this, and they made the most of the land's riches as they turned wilderness into farmland.

In the beginning, a farm produced only enough food for the family that lived on it. Soon, farmers raised a little extra to sell in town and city markets, but even city-dwellers kept chickens, pigs and kitchen gardens. In general, whatever the environment or the local farmers could not produce, the people did not eat.

Later, people were economically able to specialize. Farm families could get their clothing and staples from town and devote more time to producing more food for the local area. With westward settlement and improved transportation, farmers and ranchers were able to control bigger tracts of land to supply greater numbers of people.

But the American diet was still largely limited by season and locality, for there were no good ways to preserve most foods for very long, or to ship them very far.

Canning as a means of food preservation was developed for wide-scale practical use shortly after the Civil War, and mechanical refrigeration soon followed. These techniques made nutritious food available year round in most parts of the country. But agriculture as a business still remained small and diversified.

Then came the technological revolution. Beginning in the early decades of this century, a number of innovations combined to turn small farming into big business. Power-driven tractors and other equipment made it possible for one farmer to plant and harvest larger and larger acreages. Trucks, trains, planes and advanced refrigeration techniques allowed food to be transported over greater and greater distances. Scientifically bred seed and livestock produced higher and higher yields. Chemical fertilizers, specialized animal feed, pesticides and growth hormones increased productivity still further.

During this century, American agricultural production has risen sharply, while the number of farmers has decreased dramatically. In 1940 one farmer supplied food for twelve people; in 1975 a single farmer could feed fifty people.

Such productivity is useful, because our growing population lives increasingly in and around cities, so more people must rely on others for their food. America has also become the "breadbasket of the world," as U.S. farm exports supply an international market.

Technology has also changed the nature of farming. Once farms in an area supplied all of the different types of food—meat, produce, grain and dairy products—for that region. Today, farmers specialize. A fruit grower raises one basic kind of fruit, a wheat grower raises only wheat, a cattle rancher only cattle and so on. Rapid transportation and advanced preservation and processing techniques have made such specialization possible. But the same technology has also made huge specialized farms *necessary*.

Technology is expensive. To justify the enormous cost of buying and fueling the machines, a farmer must be able to make full use of them. They must be kept busy most of the time, bringing in a crop big enough to pay for the machines and for the new seeds and chemicals. Different crops require different machines, so the push is toward specialization. And, with the increasing complexity of the food business, a farmer may now be as expert in stocks, international trade and commodity futures as in soil and seed.

DOWN AT THE PLANT

To sell a large output, a big producer needs a big market. And that's where the food-processing industry comes in.

Thirty years ago, a "processed food" meant a can of tomatoes or a loaf of store-bought bread. Frozen foods were not introduced commercially until after World War II. And when farming was largely small and regional, so was processing. A local cannery would process all of one area's produce and distribute it to nearby stores. In some places, this system still operates. Milk especially, and some meats, don't travel too far. But meat-processing is becoming more centralized and small local plants are now often owned by large national companies.

In general, processing plants have now grown into huge automated factories that specialize in handling one type of food, which is then shipped in vast quantities across the country. Because one factory can process billions of beans or tons of tuna fish, the plant owners want to buy in huge quantities from the largest producers possible.

In some cases, growers ship a crop to a central marketplace, where packers bargain for it through brokers. But to increase productivity and efficiency, companies prefer to control as much of their particular operation as possible. Many processors own the land that produces their crop, so that they can plant the best type of seed for their operation. Or they may contract with a grower or rancher and specify or even provide the seed, feed and growing and harvesting techniques best suited to their purposes.

The chemists, engineers, biologists and other experts needed to supply technical know-how become part of the processor's staff, constantly working to improve productivity. This kind of organization requires money, so most companies process a variety of foods and other products. In many cases, food companies own or control the trucks that ship their goods, the chemical plants that produce fertilizer and pesticides, even the companies that manufacture the containers.

The food network—from farmer to grocery clerk —employs about 30 percent of the nation's work force. It also supports many other industries: the producers of feed and fertilizer, the manufacturers of advanced planting and harvesting equipment, makers of automated plant machinery, truck builders and tire manufacturers, can producers and their ore mines, carton manufacturers and their timberland. A blighted corn crop or a dried-up wheat harvest can thus deprive countless other companies and individuals of work. And this is only the *production* end of the food industry. Distribution and sales, and all the businesses that depend on them, are billion-dollar operations in themselves.

THE LONG TRIP THROUGH THE MIDDLE

Even when it's snug in a can, jar or box, our food isn't finished. It still must travel from the processor to our table, and this is usually a complex and time-consuming journey.

Most of the products on our supermarket shelves, even those that have been locally produced, have probably gone from a shipper to a distributor to a wholesaler and then to the market's warehouse before they reach the store. Some very large store chains, like A&P and Safeway, buy direct from the manufacturer and ship straight to the stores. But most items of our diet have spent days, weeks or even months in various warehouses, trucks, trains and ships before they reach the store.

THE SELLING POINT

Sales of groceries amounted to over $143 billion in 1975. Most of those sales occurred in supermarkets, and most of those supermarkets were part of a chain owned by one of a relatively few national or regional companies.

We have big grocery stores in part because we have mass food production. It is simpler and more economical if both buyer and seller can transact in bulk than if many small orders must be packed, shipped and handled. But small shopkeepers can't afford the bulk orders necessary to buy direct from the manufacturer. They must make their purchases from a wholesaler, which adds to the cost of their food. So the neighborhood grocery store must usually charge more for the same items than the chain stores. As a result many small grocery stores have closed or sold out to the chains.

Every community still has its locally owned corner grocery or general store, of course, because they can provide a kind of convenience and service that no supermarket can match. The customer is the key to the survival of both types of store, but the tendency is for the small shop to focus on what the customer wants, while the supermarket is more concerned with what it can make the customer buy. There's a big difference between the two approaches.

SEVEN
THE CHECK-OUT COUNTER

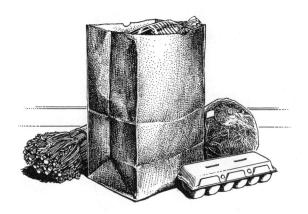

People stop in the corner grocery store when they want to buy specific items—a candy bar, a quart of milk, a loaf of bread. People go to the supermarket to do their weekly shopping and usually they leave with more than they intended to buy.

THE POWER OF SUGGESTION

A supermarket is designed to make the shopper *want* to buy. Using advertisements, sale posters or promotional gimmicks, it entices customers to come in and look around.

Inside, most supermarkets are laid out in ways that encourage people to continue walking through them. They may have music or carpeting or special lighting effects—anything that induces a trancelike state. Their shelves are arranged in part for the convenience of the shopper, but mostly to stimulate purchasing. "Modernizing" techniques like the "universal product code" and automated check-out counters give the impression of creating greater efficiency for the sake of consumer satisfaction, but they help the store more than they do the shopper.

It's fun to go shopping, even for groceries. As prices rise, we may not enjoy it as much as we once did, but shopping is still something that we tend to think of as entertaining. We enjoy a stroll along the supermarket aisles, looking at all the packages, and, of course, buying a few. The name of the game is "turnover." Only by turning over, or clearing out, the merchandise often enough is a supermarket able to get its chunk of food-industry profit.

WINNING THE VOTE

What you buy makes an impact all the way along the food network, because when you make a purchase, you are in effect casting a vote for that item. The more votes, the more sales; and the greater the profit, the happier everyone is along the line.

The supermarket doesn't care what you buy (except that some items carry a higher "profit margin" than others), as long as you buy *something*. But the food manufacturers care very much about winning as many votes as possible. So they campaign hard, and as long as they don't lie outright about their products, almost any technique qualifies as fair practice.

Packaging is designed to catch your eye and appeal to your appetite.

Shelf space is fought over, for a certain item in one spot on a particular shelf will sell better than the same item placed elsewhere. Often, company salespeople or route delivery drivers shelve their own products, pushing out the competition in the process.

Salespeople receive incentives and bonuses for surpassing their sales quotas, so they do their best to convince the store manager to give preference to their company's products.

Deals between individual salespeople and managers, or between food companies and chains, result in one brand's having better shelf space or a lower price than another. Some of these deals are legal; some are not.

Promotional devices such as contests, coupons, special sales or premiums attract customers to one brand instead of another.

Market research determines what customers want, or what they can be persuaded to buy. Market researchers call themselves the "consumers' best advocates," but they are also effective in expanding corporate sales.

Advertising is often crucial to sales. A good ad can make you buy one box of crackers instead of another, even if the unadvertised cracker tastes better and costs less.

You may have noticed that none of these competitive techniques has anything to do with the taste, quality, or nutritive value of the food involved. But they all have a lot to do with *selling* the food, and selling is what the food business is all about.

THE ONLY GAME IN TOWN

One obvious way to win the most "votes" is to be the only candidate in the race. If a bread manufacturer could operate all the bakeries in the country, people would have no choice but to buy that brand of bread. But it is next to impossible (it is *not* impossible) to achieve such a complete monopoly because of laws encouraging competition and preventing restraint of trade. Even so, the major food companies have managed to become "oligopolies" by cornering a tremendous share of a particular market.

If a large company cannot create a monopoly or even an oligopoly, it may form a conglomerate. A gigantic bakery might buy or control a dairy, a jam company, a slaughterhouse, a ketchup bottler, a pickle producer and a vegetable grower. You could buy your breakfast, lunch and dinner from the same company. Of course, the brand names would be different, so you might not even realize that all your "votes" were going to the same candidate.

Consolidated Foods, for instance, owns Sara Lee bakeries, Shasta soft drinks, Kahn's meats and Popsicles, among other brands. From General Foods you can buy Jell-O, Post cereals, Birdseye vegetables, Gaines dog food, Kool-Aid and a host of other products. United Brands markets Morrell meats, Interharvest produce and Chiquita bananas. Some of the world's largest industrial conglomerates also own famous food labels. ITT (formerly the International Telephone and Telegraph Company) owns Wonder Bread, Morton frozen foods, Hostess baked goods and others of our most popular foods.

Some food producers get us where we live, play and work, as well as where we eat. Electrolux, Fuller Brush, Gant shirts and Tyco trains are all subsidiaries of Consolidated Foods. When you munch

Fritos and sip Pepsi after playing tennis with a Wilson racquet, you're making use of products from Pepsico, which also owns a fleet of rental trucks. The Fisher-Price and Simplex toys little kids play with are all made by Quaker Oats, the "cereal company." Kenner Toys is a member of the "General Mills Fun Group."

Most food companies also include "institutional" divisions, which pack and ship products specially designed for schools, hospitals, industrial cafeterias or restaurants. Some of the big companies own restaurants, as well. General Foods owns Burger Chef, for example; Pet Foods owns Stuckey's; Pillsbury owns Burger King. So a single food supplier can own or control the raw materials, the packaging and the shipping network for its products, as well as some of the places where those products are sold.

This kind of "diversification" is good for a company since it doesn't have to put all its eggs in one basket. But a sound business practice can be less than sound for the consumer because it cuts down on competition. True competition keeps food quality higher and prices lower.

A NEW TASTE SENSATION

Crunchy Bean, Inc., which we invented back in Chapter 5, has become a conglomerate; it sells a lot more than beans. One way CBI keeps growing is by creating new products that will increase its share of the family food budget. Today it's an instant soufflé mix—an airy gourmet concoction in a box. Let's see how this new taste sensation gets from an imaginary drawing board into an imaginary mouth.

CBI's new-products development staff notices that people seem to go in for gourmet cooking, but that they still want convenience and ease of preparation. What could be better than an instant soufflé mix? The market-research staff gathers data from surveys and questionnaires distributed in a sample market area and decides that the idea is a good one.

Food technologists in the research department report that they could produce such a mix at a cost of twenty-five cents a package. CBI bookkeepers add up the cost of production, the price of advertising, distribution, salaries and general overhead, and conclude that if the soufflé is to bring the company a profit, it must sell at least a million packages initially at a price of ninety-nine cents.

While the technologists are creating the product, the promotion staff and an advertising agency work on creating a market for it. First the mix needs a name, and the experts choose "Fluffy Lite." Soon they have prepared an advertising and promotional campaign for Fluffy Lite that will have people in our test market waiting for the mix just about the time it gets to the supermarkets. (Test markets are regions, selected on the basis of some special characteristics, in which a company tries out a product before selling it nationally.)

TV commercials will show an attractive hostess whipping up the soufflé and serving it to her glamorous guests, who are looking impressed. Some of the magazine ads will aim at making women who don't serve soufflés feel guilty and inadequate. Others will point out, politely, that even a man can make Fluffy Lite. Ads in grocery-industry magazines will stress the product's qualities as a sure seller with a high profit margin. Some of the ads will carry bargain coupons. And the sales staff will be busy lining up good display space and joint promotions with the grocery stores. There will even be in-store demonstrations, showing how easy and delicious Fluffy Lite is.

Meanwhile, back in the lab, the food technicians slave over test tubes full of Fluffy Lite's ingredients: dehydrated egg yolk, dried egg white, flour, a bit of maltose, salt and dehydrated milk solids. Depending on the flavor, they stir in imitation cheese food, dehydrated fish flakes, artificial strawberry, lemon or banana flavoring or imitation chocolate. Then they add carageenin for consistency, whey for bulk, BHA and BHT as preservatives and artificial coloring to make the mix look good.

The technicians figure out the right amount of water to add to the mixture, establish a simple procedure for its preparation. And *voila!* a soufflé not quite as good as homemade, put together from dehydrated this and artificial that. Cheap, too.

CHURNING IT OUT

Fluffy Lite is ready to go into production. An assembly line has been set up to make and pack the product. Inspectors stand ready at various points to check random boxes. The factory room is glistening and spotless; CBI runs a clean shop. They can't be sure, of course, that their egg and milk suppliers are as careful, but they try to buy the best available at the price they can afford.

In almost no time, one hundred thousand packs of Fluffy Lite are ready for shipment to the test market. A new product is launched!

But what's this? Fluffy Lite isn't selling as well as predicted. People seem to be cashing in their introductory coupons and not coming back for more.

The market-research staff goes out again. They report that consumers like the idea and the taste, but it's too easy. They want to feel they've done more than pour in water and turn on the oven. So CBI takes out the dehydrated egg. The technologists adjust the formula, and new labels are printed:

"New! Improved! Add Your Own Real Fresh Eggs!"

Fluffy Lite goes back onto the market, at no reduction in price, of course, and it does so well it's being sold nationally in a few months.

Then another soufflé mix reaches the market. It tastes a little better than CBI's, and costs a few cents less, but its manufacturer does not have the promotional resources to push it, so Fluffy Lite takes over the market.

TURNED-OFF HEADS

In defense of consumers who buy such pointless and expensive convenience foods, it must be said that modern advertising, promotional and marketing techniques are almost irresistible.

From the time we're old enough to sit up, we stare glassy-eyed at the TV, where we learn that "Monster Munchies" or whatever are good for us and sweet and yummy, too. You have probably been so bombarded by TV food ads that you aren't even aware that you don't really need these costly, worthless products. Starting at an early age, you are programmed to respond to ads for "new taste sensations."

Of course, we don't have to turn off our minds when we turn on the TV, but we do. We don't have to buy any of the thousands of products on the market that do nothing for us but lighten our pockets, but we do. We don't have to assume that the government and the manufacturers will make sure everything is safe and good for us, but we do.

Even if we don't buy things like Fluffy Lite, we pay for them when prices of a company's other products are raised to meet the cost of developing a new taste treat and to cushion the profits if a new idea flops. In a big, complex and interrelated system, that's the way it is.

BIGGER AND BETTER?

In theory, we should benefit from bigness. And, up to a point, we do. Large-scale agribusiness does make available a quantity and variety of food unmatched in any other country or at any other time. Industry-sponsored research, though carried on to increase profits, has resulted in new forms of agriculture and food preservation that have enhanced our diet.

Bigness should also reduce the price we pay for our food. It is cheaper for one farmer to raise the wheat we need than for a dozen of them to do it. It's cheaper for one plant to mill the flour, bake and ship the bread than for three separate companies to do it. It is cheaper for one chain to buy carloads of merchandise than for two dozen small stores to buy in parcels. So it should be cheaper for the consumer to buy the finished product. That's the way it should work, and sometimes that's the way it does.

But when bigness gets out of hand, it works against the consumer. When agribusiness and food conglomerates grow as large as many of them have in America, they become more concerned with sales and profits than with quality and nutrition. They focus on the *means* of production and marketing rather than on the *end* of providing valuable food. When a few giant corporations dominate a given market, competition is restricted. Limited competition works against us by narrowing our choices.

There are other reasons, too, why we end up paying more for our food. As growing and processing become ever more centralized, food must travel a very long and complicated route to the store. None of the participants in the food network works for free. The shipper, the distributor, the wholesaler, the salespeople, the advertisers, the supermarkets and all the brokers and warehousers in between have their own expenses and they need to make a profit. So the price advantage the consumer might have gained from the cost-saving mass-production techniques is lost by the time the middlemen have taken their cut. In fact, *sixty cents* of every food dollar goes for packaging, transportation, advertising, supermarket overhead and other nonnutritional expenditures. The farmer gets an average of twenty-three cents of our food dollar.

EIGHT
FARMER SAM

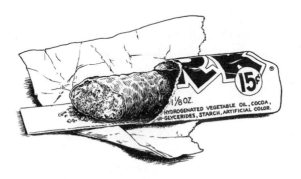

If you knew that a twenty-cent candy bar cost the manufacturer next to nothing for sugar, artificial chocolate flavoring and additives, you might feel cheated. But you probably don't think about that when you buy the candy. Few of us do. And that's the problem: just as most of us eat without thinking, we also buy without thinking.

Twentieth-century Americans have come to rely on Uncle Sam to do much of their food thinking for them. The federal government has an obvious interest in guaranteeing the purity of the food we eat and in insuring a continuing food supply for all of us. Through its various agencies, it tries to be consumer's advocate, middleman's watchdog and farmer's friend while regulating the flow of foods and funds toward a goal of political balance and economic stability.

It's a big job, and one that would take more than one book to describe in detail. Here's a quick look at how Farmer Sam helps keep our bellies full.

TOWARD PURITY, PRODUCTIVITY AND FAIRNESS

The federal government first began to play a major role in the business of food back around the turn of the century, when the business was just beginning to get big. Early food processing was unsanitary, and early food processors were often unscrupulous, so the government drafted laws designed to protect the consumer from being sold impure food.

Today the food-supply network is vast, and the government maintains an equally vast bureaucracy to try to police it. Congress conducts periodic investigations into national agricultural policy, nutrition status and food safety, and passes laws designed to correct defects. State and local departments of health regulate those food products which do not fall under federal authority. But the great majority of food crosses state lines, so thousands of federal employees devote millions of working hours to food.

KEEPING IT CLEAN: The U.S. Department of Agriculture (USDA) is responsible for inspecting crops, livestock and processing facilities and grading much of our food.

The U.S. Public Health Service sets standards for sanitation and watches out for food-borne illnesses.

The Food and Drug Administration (FDA) determines which of the countless additives and processing techniques are safe, and bans those it considers dangerous.

The National Academy of Sciences establishes nutritional needs and recommends methods of providing for them.

KEEPING IT HONEST: The Federal Trade Commission (FTC) regulates advertising, marketing and other business practices in an effort to keep them fair and honest.

The Office of Consumer Affairs is charged with representing consumer interests, even when they conflict with the policies of other government agencies.

The FDA joins with the FTC to make sure that food products are honestly labeled.

MAKING IT WORK: USDA research develops new

plant strains, animal breeds, fertilizers and pesticides to increase production, and USDA agents advise farmers on how to make best use of their land.

The Department of Health, Education and Welfare and other agencies work on ways to improve the healthfulness and nutritional value of the foods we eat.

LETTING US KNOW: Most federal agencies and many state and local departments that deal with food have "offices of communications" that publish a wide variety of material about their findings and activities. The USDA is an especially good source of information about food production, preparation, storage and needs (see pages 130–136).

HELPING US OUT: For those citizens who cannot get enough to eat, the government provides help through operations like the food-stamp program and school feeding projects.

TOWARD A BALANCE

As you know by now, food is much more than just something to eat. Food is central to the political and economic life of the country, as well. Since the food business makes up such a substantial portion of our national economy, the government must take an interest in the financial costs and benefits. For example, the government helps farmers maintain their incomes. It buys a lot of food for its own use, and it also buys food it doesn't use. To help farmers keep their prices high enough for adequate profits, the government may buy up a surplus so that a commodity doesn't flood the market and lower growers' incomes or cause them to reduce output, which would eventually create scarcity and higher prices. Uncle Sam has at times paid farmers *not* to grow food, since that was less expensive than buying and storing surpluses.

The government must also attempt to keep the price of food low enough for people to buy it. Official means of achieving this goal vary with the administration and the circumstances. Price controls, such as those imposed during the Nixon administration, are a direct means of keeping food costs down. One indirect method is the Justice Department's power to enforce antitrust laws. These laws are designed to insure competition by preventing price-fixing and monopolistic businesses.

Food is a political issue, too. The people who grow the food, the people who manufacture and distribute it, the people who eat it and the people who haven't enough food to eat are all voters. Their representatives in Congress and in the executive branch must take them into consideration in the regulation of our food supply. Policies and legislation that please one group may anger another. Balancing all their needs and wants is an important part of the American political process.

DOES IT WORK?

The governing of food is at least as complicated as the matter of food itself. But does it work? We've come to take for granted the government's contribution to the food network, and many of us assume that Uncle Sam is always reliable and unbiased. But now people are beginning to wonder if he can handle the job.

Food-stamp and school meal programs have praiseworthy goals, but some experts complain that too little attention is paid to the nutritional content of food supplied by these projects.

USDA grades also ignore the nutritional value of the foods they rate. Many people believe that when they buy "fancy" produce or Grade A eggs and chickens, they are buying the best and freshest food, but they aren't; they are just buying the *best-looking* food. The USDA grades rate food primarily on its appearance. A Grade B egg, for instance, is just as fresh and nutritious as a Grade A egg; Grade A just looks prettier when it's fried. "Fancy" produce is just that: fancy—good-looking but not necessarily tastier or more wholesome than lower-grade fruits and vegetables. Some consumer advocates argue that if the government is going to grade foods at all, it should grade them for their nutritional quality rather than for their outward appearance.

Other arguments rage over whether Uncle Sam is as even-handed as he's supposed to be. Food-inspection and -protection laws were passed to protect the consumer. But in practice, these laws often seem to benefit the producer by allowing ingredients, grading standards and labeling practices that serve more to confuse than to protect. The food industry can influence the government by lobbying for its causes. Critics say that the regulatory system operates unfairly because representatives respond to those who can lobby the hardest, and lobbying takes the kind of money that big corporations have and small farmers and consumers lack.

Industry executives can also exert a more subtle influence by joining the staffs of agencies that regulate the same corporations they came from and by then rejoining industry after gaining contacts within the government. For example, Earl Butz, the secretary of agriculture, came to the USDA from the board of directors of the Ralston-Purina Company (one of the nation's largest producers of food for humans, pets and livestock). Clifford Hardin, his predecessor as agriculture secretary, took over Butz's job at Ralston-Purina. The lawyer who drafted new

FDA regulations of "imitation foods" favorable to the food industry worked for a law firm representing large food processors at the time. He then became the general counsel (chief lawyer) at the FDA, the agency charged with administering the regulations. The general counsel he replaced became head of a major food-industry group.

Critics say the government relies too heavily on the expertise of food-industry executives, at the expense of the consumer. But the government may need to rely on the experience of these people because often it hasn't the resources to develop its own experts.

WHAT WE DON'T KNOW CAN HURT US

A basic problem with government nutrition policy is that nobody knows enough about nutrition and human needs to be able to say with certainty what is good and what isn't good for all people in all cases. Nutrition is a new science. Vitamins were first discovered only about sixty-five years ago, and until the nineteenth century, no one had a clear idea of how the body used food at all. Nutrition as a science has made great strides, and we now have a pretty good idea about how much of what we need to eat, and why. But that doesn't mean that the science has discovered everything we need to know about food.

Until recently, nobody paid much attention to fiber, but it is becoming apparent that a diet lacking fiber causes problems. Nobody thought ahead of time to link food additives to emotional disorders, but now there's enough evidence to raise suspicions.

Food manufacturers maintain that they can turn out artificial foods and make them just as nutritious as the natural product by fortifying them with vitamins and minerals. But can they? Artificial orange drink may have "all the vitamin C of fresh-squeezed orange juice," but it lacks the other vitamins and minerals real fruit juice offers. Enriched white bread is said to be as nutritious as whole-wheat, but enriching restores only part of the food value, and none of the fiber, of the whole grain. As our foods increasingly become laboratory creations, food companies and government regulators should be required to exert more effort toward making them "just like the real thing," if they can achieve that goal at all.

It *seems* logical to argue that foods are chemicals and vitamins are chemicals, so a chemical compound created in a lab should serve the same purpose as the natural version. Maybe it will, but we don't really know.

By law, no artificial ingredient may be added to food unless it has been tested for safety, but there are exceptions to the rule. If the additive has been in use since 1958, it is allowed *until* it is proven to be dangerous. In an effort to make food inspection more effective, new federal standards are continuously proposed, put into effect and altered. One current standard, in use since 1958, forbids the use in food of any substance that has been shown to cause cancer in test animals. Critics of this regulation maintain that any substance given in excess can cause cancer. Other critics argue that few of the testing standards are tough enough. So not only is food safety difficult, it is also controversial.

The controversy over the dye called Red #2 is a case in point. For years, consumer groups and scientists argued that this food coloring (which was added to a wide variety of foods—even some that were not red) caused cancer. Some researchers have also linked it to a childhood disorder called hyperkinesis. The Food and Drug Administration, the agency responsible in such matters, maintained that the dye was safe, until it abruptly banned its use early in 1976. Food manufacturers went to court in an unsuccessful effort to overturn the ban—all for a substance which, harmful or not, serves no useful purpose other than to make processed foods more attractive and thus more salable. Meanwhile, scientists outside of the immediate controversy noted that many of the experiments involving the safety of Red #2 were "botched," and that no matter what their actual results, the tests were alarmingly typical of the careless techniques employed by government testers.

Even when ingredients are proven unsafe, the government is often dangerously slow in banning them. For years, evidence accumulated that the artificial sweeteners called cyclamates were dangerous; the FDA acknowledged their hazard in 1969, but did not ban them from food until 1970. A growth-hormone, diethylstilbestrol (DES), is known to cause cancer in the offspring of people who ingest it, yet it is still in use. In instances like these, as in the case of Red #2, pressure from the industries that benefit from the substance is often to blame for the delay. Cyclamate production was a multimillion-dollar business before 1970.

We don't know how humans will thrive on artificial fortification until we have tried it for a long time. And we don't know what undiscovered ingredient in "real" foods might contribute to our health in ways the artificial compounds can't. What we don't know *can* hurt us.

Some consumers argue that we're safe only when we have more and better government regulations to protect us. Others think the whole government regulatory business should be abandoned, on the theory that people have a right to make their own mistakes. It seems more sensible to overhaul the entire system of inspection, grading and approving—to make them more appropriate to the potential dangers of today's and tomorrow's food. However, such a drastic change is probably impossible, given the bureaucratic structure that has grown up around the food-protection procedure.

WHAT ABOUT THE BIG PICTURE?

Even with that bureaucratic fortress of expertise, the government has not yet managed to establish an overall policy that would guarantee all of us a safe, economical, sufficient and continuing supply of food. In part that failure is because of the bureaucracy itself: all those offices and officers in various branches and agencies tend to compete and argue with one another. In part, it is because of practical politics.

Still, it is important that the U.S. have some kind of broad agricultural and nutritional plan. The government has an interest in keeping its own citizens nourished, now and in the future.

NINE
FOOD IS POWER

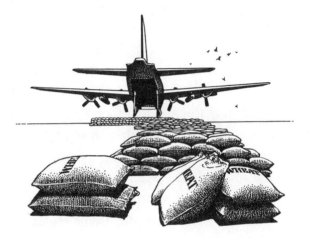

Since the beginning of civilization, food supplies have been the blue chips in the power plays between peoples and nations.

A prime goal of ancient marauding tribes was to conquer those settled societies that had a secure farming system. Later, geographically weak nations would fight to establish colonies in agriculturally productive lands. Throughout history, unfair distribution of food supplies has caused riots, wars and revolutions. And farm products have been a medium of exchange ever since people began trading: rum for sugar, cotton for tea, wool for spices—anything one country can grow for something it can't.

FOOD IS MONEY

Today the world is more complex, but it operates in the same way it always has. A small country may boast of bananas or sugar as its only national resource, but it can trade those commodities for goods and money to meet its other needs. A Middle Eastern kingdom may be rolling in oil, but it must use some of the "petrodollars" it gets from the U.S. to buy food for its desert people. America's resources for food production are virtually unequaled, and we use those resources to trade for items we lack. We rely on other nations for coffee, cocoa, sugar, spices and other staples that we can't produce, and we spend a good portion of our national income for them.

FOOD IS A WEAPON

Because food is so valuable, the United States uses it as a tool in diplomacy. The Soviet Union needs wheat, for example. We sell wheat to the USSR, and in return we expect "détente" and accommodations in international activities. We sell wheat to China, and hope that this sale will make the Chinese less hostile toward us. Someday a weak, hungry nation may develop an atomic bomb, and, by agreement, refrain from using it in return for food for its population.

Food is an excellent weapon. When the government of an underdeveloped country proposes policies that the U.S. feels are threatening, we can cut off food aid or trade. In the past, it was the people with food who won the wars. Today, it may be the people with the food who prevent them.

BELLIES, FAT AND SWOLLEN

Diplomats may think of food as a weapon, but most people don't. Few of the hungry in the world today think of food in terms of war and peace, petrodollars or détente. They are simply hungry, and they want to eat.

The population of the world is growing too rapidly to keep up with its food supply, and it's growing fastest in the areas where food is scarcest. What's going to happen? That depends on how the nations of the world manage the earth's food and resources for production. For now, people starve.

Humanity has always known starvation, but today there are more people around to suffer from it, and more sophisticated ways of letting the rest of the world know about it than ever before. During the first modern world food crisis of the 1970s, some experts alarmingly predicted that the entire earth would soon run out of food. Now it seems that, with wise management, humanity will have enough food, *if* we distribute it in such a way that all of us are fed.

THE LIFEBOAT

One way to make sure that there is enough food to go around is to get rid of some of the people who eat it. If the rich nations simply do not provide food for the poorer ones, the hungry will die, and the rest of us will be able to fill ourselves.

This solution is called "triage," or "the lifeboat ethic." When a ship is sinking, those who can reach the lifeboats survive, and the rest drown—or, in this case, starve. Not only is such a proposal immoral, but it is also impractical. Desperate swimmers can tip over a lifeboat in their efforts to board it, and drown all the occupants. Starving nations can explode nuclear bombs or blow up oil wells, plantations and mineral mines.

A more responsible method of making sure that everyone has enough to eat is to reduce population growth. Birth-control programs are an essential part of any food distribution or nutritional improvement effort, but they are often very difficult to carry out. The people who need birth control the most have difficulty accepting the reasons for it. Some cultures place a high status on having large families. Many other people have become accustomed to having some of their children die young, so they have many children with the hope that a few will survive to adulthood.

There would also be more food available if we wasted less. American tastes, food habits and beliefs about nutrition have contributed greatly to the problem of inadequate world food supplies. We have come to like packaged breakfast cereals and meat fattened on grain. The amount of grain that goes into our breakfasts or our steak dinners could feed a lot of hungry people.

We've compounded the problem by exporting our eating habits to other people around the world. The Soviet Union has acquired our taste for grain-fed beef, so in the last few years they needed to buy grain from us to feed their cattle, and have used up that much more of the world's grain reserves.

SHARING THE WEALTH

Another method of insuring an adequate food supply is for the world to share its food more equally. As a result of the food crisis of 1974, a World Food Council was established to oversee international supplies and manage any future crises. A world food bank has also been proposed. This "bank" would hold reserves of surplus food, which in an emergency could be dispensed to hungry peoples. But many doubt that such an apparently sensible share-the-food project would actually be put into practice, because food is such an important source of income and political power.

Since World War II, the United States has prided itself on its programs to feed the hungry. It is true that by shipping our surpluses overseas, we have prevented a lot of people from starving. Such programs have also encouraged less productive nations to become dependent upon us for food. But when we cannot afford to share our food because of a poor harvest or other reasons, these countries have no agricultural resources of their own to fall back on.

Many U.S. farmers object to growing surpluses for shipment overseas. They feel that they could earn more for their crops if foreigners bought them at current market prices, rather than having the U.S. government buying at lower, fixed rates. Farmers' groups have urged the government to help poorer nations develop their industrial and financial resources so that citizens of those countries could buy American agricultural products. But this kind of project takes time, and the government seems to be just as happy to buy up surpluses and ship them overseas to win friends and influence people.

EXPORTING EXPERTISE

If we are unwilling to give food away, perhaps we can at least teach the less-developed countries how to grow their own food. But there are hazards even in this approach.

In the past, our tendency has been to think that a technique that works in this country will work everywhere else if we just put enough money and effort into it. Government and corporate experts have gone around the world modernizing agriculture along American lines. But the system requires vast areas of land, highly advanced tools, sophisticated chemicals and a strong economic and technological network to back it up. Farmers in Asia, Africa or South America may learn how to work a tractor, but that does them little good if they can't afford the fuel to run it. Chemical fertilizers and pesticides may increase production dramatically, but they are expensive and often in short supply.

A poor nation has to upgrade and revolutionize its entire social, economic and technological structure to support western-style farming, or it has to learn how to improve agricultural yields using the tools and resources it currently has available.

Experts from government agencies, private corporations and international organizations have lately taken the latter approach. They focus on practical

ways to help small farmers with limited resources
find new crops and productive ways of growing
them within their social system. Such techniques of
international assistance and cooperation should
prove effective in the long run. Unfortunately, the
world may have only a short time in which to produce the food. A combination of all the suggested
methods will be needed to avert another major food
crisis.

SO WHAT?

A major world food shortage would affect all the
inhabitants of planet earth, not just the poor nations. The earth's resources are limited, and made
more so by our growing population and wasteful
habits. If we are to avoid going down with the ship,
nations will have to find ways to protect those resources and to make the most efficient use of them,
wherever they might be.

What can *you* do about international food problems? The most important thing you can do right
now is to think about them. Think about what you
would do if you were in charge. If you can change
your head, you can change your habits. You may
have to change your habits before you're much
older.

There may come a time when what you eat is not

simply a moral matter but a practical problem. If the politicians succeed in establishing an international food-sharing system, you will be able to feed a hungry family by giving up some of your portion of grain. If the politicians fail, the world may well run out of food.

TEN
THE NEXT COURSE

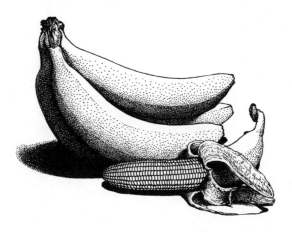

If you are going to have enough to eat during your lifetime, humanity will have to find and invent new sources of nutrition and make better use of the world's current food resources.

SUPERCORN!

One approach to the problem of dwindling food is to find ways to yield more nutrition per acre. Modern agriculture has been working at this for years by strengthening fertilizers, inventing new machines and crossbreeding plants and animals for higher production. Now, the need is greater, the land is scarcer and the time is shorter.

So far, the efforts have met with some success. In the early 1970s, the earth seemed to be on the brink of a "green revolution." New strains of "miracle rice" had been developed that would increase yield dramatically, so that a country like India could produce more food without having to cultivate more land. High-yielding varieties of wheat, fantastically productive and resistant to disease, promised great results. "High-lysine" corn produced ears that were more nutritious and abundant than the old-fashioned kind.

But, the optimism dimmed when it appeared that these superplants fulfilled their promise only when they were raised under exacting, well-controlled conditions, using expensive and increasingly scarce chemical fertilizers. People in the poor countries who were supposed to reap the benefits of these supercrops lacked the skill and the funds to raise them. Improved plants are yielding improved results, but the "revolution" is not yet upon us.

NITROGEN TRAPS

Some plants, like clover, alfalfa, peanuts and most peas and beans, are capable of "trapping" nitrogen from the air and "fixing" it in the soil. Since nitrogen is an essential part of protein, these plants serve as an excellent source of protein for humans and animals. The Food and Agriculture Organization of the United Nations and other agencies are searching for new plants that can be developed as crops to produce alternate sources of protein.

Nitrogen is also excellent fertilizer. Scientists are now working to harness the power of known nitrogen traps, and to transfer this ability to other types of plants. In that way, they hope to expand the world's fertilizer supply and decrease the dependence on expensive chemical compounds.

NEWFANGLED FOODS

The USDA and other researchers are studying ways to make meat healthier and more nutritious by breeding animals that are both meatier and lower in fat. Efforts are being made to improve grazing land, so that more herds can be raised on grass. Agricultural scientists are also developing miniature fruit trees and tiny vegetable plants that could yield large harvests in small spaces.

In addition to the improvement of old crops, the search is on for totally new sources of nutrition. Researchers are testing a variety of plants that have never been food crops, but that could provide nutrition for humans and animals.

The sea is the earth's largest untapped resource. Already, fish species like the krill, not normally eaten by humans, are being harvested and processed into flour that provides a protein-rich supplement. Animals like the manatee, never thought of as livestock, may also be a part of our diets in the future. Marine biologists are studying other forms of sea life as protein sources. Kelp, or seaweed, has long been a part of the diet of island peoples and their livestock. Now food experts realize that seaweed and algae, as well as yeasts and fungi, can yield high-quality protein. Soon these products may be introduced on a wider scale.

WASTE NOT

We waste more than we realize. For years, food processors discarded everything not needed for their products. Whey, for example, is a byproduct of the cheese manufacturing process. Until recently, whey was dumped into the most convenient river, creating pollution. Then someone realized that whey is an excellent source of protein. Now at least one dairy company reclaims the whey and markets it as a protein-rich food supplement and healthful additive. At home we throw away bones and vegetable peelings that could make nourishing soup stock. Instead of saving and reheating uneaten foods, we call them "leftovers" and turn up our noses.

We even waste our waste. Animal (and in some places, human) excrement has been the most common fertilizer for centuries. But today, many farmers pay for chemical fertilizers and get rid of the cow manure. It may not be as potent as chemicals, but it makes more sense to spread it around than to throw it away. Some companies buy manure and "sterilize" it for gardening use, and one researcher has even found a way to process manure so that it can be used as animal feed. Animals can also be fed from algae raised on the sludge left over after petroleum is refined. "Waste" can be put to good use.

OUT OF THE TEST TUBE

While some scientists are working in the field, others are working in the lab. You've been eating "laboratory foods" for a long time without thinking twice about it. Labs produce the chemicals that fertilize crops, kill pests and spur animal growth, of course. In labs, scientists learned to concentrate orange juice, dehydrate vegetables or fortify milk, and made the countless other discoveries that contribute to our diet.

Food is also being created in laboratories. The "chocolate" on the last candy bar you ate was probably produced from raw cotton. The cheese on your cheese sandwich was probably a "cheese food" made from a powder. Imitation eggs claim to offer the nutrition and taste of eggs without the cholesterol content and without much help from a chicken. New foods like these are forerunners of lab products that could be valuable additions to the world's food supply. By some estimates, fabricated foods may make up 80 percent of the American diet by 1985.

But while the need for food is urgent, so is the need for safe and valuable food. If we are to increase our intake of artificial foods, new methods may be needed to insure their nutritional worth. Let's hope the food industry and government regulators will proceed with greater caution when introducing new foods than they have in the past.

EAT WITH YOUR HEAD

Recycled foods, test-tube foods—how will you ever manage to swallow all that?

Don't worry, you probably won't be eating your squiggly green sea creatures raw. They will have been converted into flour or some other more appetizing food. If you eat packaged meat extenders, bacon-flavored bits or imitation sausage, you're already eating soy protein that's been converted into familiar forms, so what else is new?

And never fear, if you can pay the price, you will always be able to have a juicy steak and fresh fruits and vegetables, and as many sweets and snacks as you want. But they'll be expensive, because they will be increasingly costly to produce. Some farmers are already switching to grain-growing, because raising fruits and vegetables is not profitable enough. Many livestock producers have gone out of business because meat doesn't bring them a good return on their investment.

If you think of yourself as a creature of habit and you can't imagine yourself eating any of those "weird" foods, think again. Your food habits have already changed a lot in your lifetime. You probably love some foods you hated when you were little, and vice versa. And you're probably eager to try a "new taste sensation" that the manufacturer has created by turning potato powder into a newfangled potato chip. So you're more adaptable than you thought.

In the future, you will have to be even more adaptable. And if you're to stay healthy you'll have to eat as much with your head as with your mouth. You will have to know a lot about basic nutrition to be able to select a diet that's good for you. And you'll need to be able to choose wisely from among the various new foods that the processing labs turn out.

ELEVEN

TRYING IT ON FOR TASTE

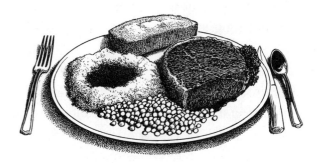

The "ideal" American dinner is steak, chicken or roast beef served with plenty of gravy, potatoes, vegetables, bread, butter and dessert. For most people, a day's menu would not be complete without meat at least once a day and usually more often, some kind of packaged or frozen pastry, an instant side dish or other mix, vegetables and fruits (fresh, frozen or canned), soda pop and lots of snacks. We're so used to our daily diets that it's hard to imagine eating any other way. But there are other food patterns that work just as well, and some even make more sense than ours.

People in an island nation like Japan eat mainly fish and seafood, rice, soy and other bean products, seaweeds and a few green vegetables. The Chinese customarily eat almost no beef, but build a menu from a little pork, poultry or fish, rice, soy products and a variety of vegetables.

People in Latin America can afford to eat almost no meat, but their staple dish, rice and beans, is an equally good source of protein. Tribesmen of North Africa and the Near East get an adequate diet from whole grains, beans, seeds and milk products supplemented by dates and other fruits. Plenty of peasants have survived for centuries on potatoes, bread, cabbage, milk and cheese, a diet that can provide all the essential nutrients. Some cultures eat insects, which may offend Western tastes, but bugs are a good source of protein. And a totally vegetarian diet, whether followed from religious convictions, personal principles or economic necessity, can provide all a person needs for health.

Throughout the world, and throughout history, people have managed to select nutritious diets from a variety of foods, so that humankind was able to thrive before anyone knew about vitamins, minerals or rare roast beef.

THE FOOD CHAIN

When you come right down to it, we get all of our

food from the sun. Plants use energy from the sun for photosynthesis, the process by which they combine carbon dioxide (CO_2) from the air and water (H_2O) from the earth into carbohydrates (CH_2O). Animals eat the plants and convert their carbohydrates into stored fat and muscle protein. We eat the plants and animals, and make our own conversion of the sun's energy.

This cycle is called a food chain. A small fish eats microscopic sea organisms; then it is eaten by a larger fish, which in turn is eaten by a human. In another food chain, a steer is fattened on feed made from corn and soybean plants, and then is fed to us. Experts have estimated that it takes sixteen pounds of corn and soybeans to produce one pound of steak.

To eat "low on the food chain" means to eat products that are closer to the beginning of the chain (the soybeans, for example) than to its end (the steer). You can get the same amount of protein found in a pound of steak from only a half-pound of soybeans, and at a much lower cost. But you don't have to trade in your steak for soybeans to get complete nutrition.

TRADITIONAL MENUS

For nutrition and taste, there's nothing wrong with a traditional "American" meal. Spaghetti with tomato sauce and cheese, bread and salad is just as nutritious as a steak or a juicy roast-beef dinner. A dinner of fried rice, seafood, bean sprouts and stir-fried vegetables serves the same purpose. A meal of rice, tortillas, black beans and peppers offers completely adequate nutrition.

Greens with "potlikker" (the water the greens are cooked in, which contains much of their vitamins and minerals), corn bread and bacon can be as good for the body as they are for the soul. The traditional Boston baked beans with brown bread needs only a vegetable to make it a nutritionally complete meal. Even a peanut-butter sandwich is nutritionally valuable if it's made with whole-wheat bread and eaten with milk and carrot and celery sticks. And a "leftovers" supper of homemade soup, bread and cheese can be as good for you as a four-square Sunday dinner.

We get ourselves into nutritional trouble when we eat over-processed versions of these meals. Our meat has been raised on growth hormones and overly fattened. The bread has had the fiber and most of the vitamins refined out of it (some, but not all of the vitamins are replaced in "enriched" breads). We often substitute dehydrated soups or watery, canned stews for the homemade variety. We overindulge in refined sugar and don't get enough of the fruits that provide vitamins along with their sweetness. We eat rice that has had the nutrition "polished" off of it. We eat "Mexican" or "Chinese" food from a mix instead of making it from fresh ingredients. We eat food that has been preserved, treated and colored with artificial substances.

At home we over-process food ourselves: we throw out the nutritious liquid from our canned goods and we usually overcook fresh produce; we fill up on starchy and sugary snacks that offer nothing but calories and crunch; and we wash it all down with a cola that gives us nothing but fizz and cavities.

HEALTH FOODS

Some people hope to avoid the pitfalls of the standard menu by turning to "health foods." Health foods can be exotic and expensive items purchased from a special health-food store, or they can be a more traditional food raised without chemical assistance and processed as little as possible.

You may think of a health-food diet as consisting of yogurt, wheat germ, honey and little else, but if you ate "natural foods" you wouldn't necessarily be eating much differently than you do today. Your bread and cereal would be made from whole grains rather than refined flours. Your vegetables would be fresh or processed without added ingredients. Your sweets would be fruits or home-baked pastries rather than candy and store-bought cakes. You might snack on nuts and juice instead of chips and soda. And most of your food would be cooked at home rather than produced at a factory and pre-served and processed with chemical additives.

Home-cooked foods or "natural" meals offer several advantages over the increasingly typical American menu. They usually cost less than processed foods. They are lower in fat and higher in vitamins and fiber so they are healthier than a packaged dinner. "Natural" meals tend to come from lower on the food chain than a meal heavy in meat.

Of course, meat can be a useful and efficient food. Animals can eat shrubbery and grasses that humans cannot digest. They can convert that greenery into protein that humans can use. And livestock can be raised on land that will support no other crop. Meat byproducts (the inedible portions of the animal) serve a variety of industrial purposes. It is only when herds are fattened before slaughter by being fed grains that eating them becomes wasteful.

But meat is far from being our only good source of protein, as you can see from the protein equivalency chart on page 112.

TRY IT—YOU'LL LIKE IT

If you're in the habit of meat and potatoes, do yourself a favor by sampling another menu. Make your own breakfast buns from whole-wheat flour, grain, fruit and nuts. Substitute a cup of yogurt, or even a peanut-butter sandwich, for the cafeteria meal or your lunchtime candy bar. Snack on peanuts and an apple after school instead of French fries and a cola. Try some rice and beans or Chinese-style food you've fixed yourself instead of a packaged hamburger dinner. The more foods you try, the more you may find you like.

TWELVE

THINK BEFORE YOU EAT

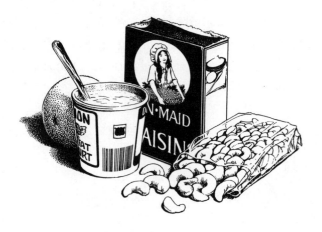

When you think before you eat, you can look better, feel better, function better and grow better. You can help make a small dent in the world's food problem. And you can hang on to some of the pocket money you're spending now for empty-calorie snacks.

Here are some suggested ways to accomplish all that without radically changing the pattern of your daily life. As you read them you'll probably come up with your own ideas.

FIGURE IT OUT: Keep a record of everything you eat for a day or two, plus when, with whom and how you felt when you ate it. While you're at it, jot down how much of your own pocket money you spend for food. Leave space to note the nutritional value of your daily diet. Then, compare your eating habits with the basic nutritional information outlined on page 108. How does what you eat stack up against what you need? What are some simple ways to improve your intake (and cut down on your expenses) without changing your lifestyle? Learn what amounts of proteins, carbohydrates, fats, vitamins and minerals you need to keep yourself at your best.

DON'T GO BANANAS: If you've read this far, you're probably someone who's concerned about the way you eat. Fine. But watch out. Don't go to the other extreme and try to subsist on phony "health foods" and fad diets. If you want to be a vegetarian, O.K. But learn enough about nonmeat protein sources so that you don't waste away. If you want to eat "organic" or "natural," do it. But don't plunge into *any* kind of diet that is not balanced. You need protein, fat, carbohydrates and all those vitamins and minerals in their proper amounts and proportions. Don't be fooled into thinking that some magic diet will solve all your problems, or that a super-supplement will make up for what you're missing.

It won't, and it *can* harm you. The best way to check out a change in your eating habits is to see your doctor, health clinic, or school's nutritionist.

DON'T EXPECT MIRACLES: You won't wake up feeling like a new person the morning after you switch from junk to good foods. Eating well is a long-term project. If you make it a lifetime habit, you will be better off than if you eat poorly, but the improvement will be so gradual that you won't notice a dramatic change.

MAKE IT SECOND NATURE: It may seem that so much thinking about food would make eating a chore. But it won't. With only a little practice, eating conscientiously will become such a habit that it will be second nature. It won't occur to you to buy a candy bar or soda when nuts and juice are available, or you won't even consider making a meal from a mix instead of from scratch. And food will still be a pleasure. Eating *should* be a pleasure. If it becomes a fetish then it can make life unpleasant for you and for those around you.

BEWARE OF POPPING PILLS: Many people believe that they need to take a daily vitamin supplement and assume that "one a day can't hurt you." But if they eat well, they don't need vitamin pills, and vitamins can hurt you. Ask your doctor before supplementing your diet with any vitamin or mineral pill, even the standard one-daily kind. And *never* dose yourself with specialized vitamins, minerals or food supplements except on the specific advice of your doctor. Unless you have some special medically diagnosed problem, a large intake of vitamins, minerals or concentrated proteins can be harmful.

DIET RIGHT: If you're a typical teen-ager, you're probably worried about gaining weight. If so, it is a good bet you need a better idea of what "dieting" is all about. Check some of the books on page 132.

If you're an athlete, you may think you need a superdiet to build your body or make you a sports star. You don't. You just need a balanced diet, reinforced with some extra calories when you're really energetic. Don't feel you must overload on proteins. And don't skimp on water when you're exercising.

START STRONG: No matter who you are, you probably need a better breakfast. That means taking in about one fourth of your day's calorie and protein requirements before you start your day's activities. It does not necessarily mean sitting down with the family for a standard breakfast-type meal. A bowl of soup, a hamburger or a plate of last night's macaroni and cheese along with some fruit, juice or milk are just as valuable as cereal or bacon and eggs. A cheese or meat sandwich will give you good nutrition if you're in a hurry—it is better for you than a candy bar or a doughnut.

SNACK SMART: Snacking itself isn't bad; it's what you snack on that does you in. You don't have to be a hermit to eat right. When you're hanging around with your friends, buy a bag of peanuts or popcorn instead of potato or corn chips. If fruit is available, that's even better. Treat yourself to an ice-cream bar or yogurt-on-a-stick instead of a frozen sugar-water pop. Have chocolate milk or a milk shake instead of a sugary soda. Pizza and hamburger are more useful ways to spend your time and money than French fries or candy.

At home, try snacking on anything but "snack foods." Cheese, peanut butter, fresh fruits and vegetables, yogurt, homemade milk shakes, whole-wheat crackers or nuts can be just as handy and just as much fun as potato chips and pretzels. Try ice water or fruit juice instead of soda pop.

HANG ON TO YOUR CASH: How much pocket money do you have at your disposal any day or week? Teenagers as a group spent $25.3 billion in 1975, and if only 10 percent of that money went for food, that's a lot of money for eating. If you use your head, you can save some of that money, and eat better, too.

A fifteen-cent bag of peanuts or popcorn instead of a twenty-cent candy bar will save you a nickel and get a bit of nourishment for your money.

But why spend anything? Take your own snacks when you go out. Peanuts you buy in bulk at the store or popcorn you've popped at home can keep your mouth busy at the movies, and they cost a lot less than the candy-stand variety. A mixture of nuts, raisins and other dried fruits tastes a lot better than vending-machine yummies, and gives you more of that "quick energy" the candy companies tout—without the empty calories.

TAKE A STAND: Hardly anyone likes the institutional food served in most school cafeterias. Students have been complaining about school food for generations. But griping about the food is one thing; doing something about it is another matter. Feeding a lot of people on a little money is difficult, so variety and flavor have generally been overlooked. But school food is supposed to be nutritious, and once you know a bit more about nutrition, you can complain if the lunch doesn't offer much food value. Get your facts straight, and propose some alternatives to the people in charge.

At the very least, you can work to improve the snacks your school makes available. If candy and crackers fill the racks at the end of the lunch line or the vending machines in your school, get organized.

A group of you could generate enough interest to have junk food replaced with nuts, fruit, yogurt, milk and other nourishing foods. Students in other schools have done it, so why not you? Some student groups have even set up their own snack-sales tables in school, to provide good snacks and raise some money at the same time.

TAKE A TASTE: Of course, you may not like the cafeteria menus simply because they're not what you're used to. The liver, carrot salad and squash offer super nutrition, but you just can't stand them. Or you *think* you can't. Did you ever try? Start small. Take a taste of something you've always thought you would hate. Maybe it's not as bad as you imagined, and it might even taste good. Break some old eating habits and add new foods to your diet. Fish, leaner meat, whole-grain foods and beans can add a lot of nutrition to your diet without adding to your family's food budget. When new products like soy sausage or fishmeal come on the market, give them a try. (A note about beans: they often cause gas and indigestion, especially in people who aren't used to eating them. Don't eat a potful at the first sitting; eat a small portion and let your body get used to the idea.)

DON'T BE FOOLED: Of course, not all new products

will be worth eating, especially those that come on with a big advertising campaign. Keep in mind that advertising is expensive. The promotion costs are either added to the product's price or subtracted from its quality, or both. If you must buy candy, for instance, you'll save money by buying a bag of candy bars bearing a supermarket's "house brand" instead of picking up a bar you've just seen on three TV commercials. (A "house brand" is a product packed specially for a supermarket chain. It may be manufactured by a "name-brand" company but it is not advertised or attractively packaged and therefore costs less. You get more product for your money.)

You don't have to be a puppet of the food manufacturers and advertisers. When people began to be interested in healthier "natural" foods, the food industry was quick to respond by turning out "natural" cereals. Not all the claims were strictly true, because many of the products were processed with additives. Also, the new items cost more than the standard varieties, but they sold anyway. Read the labels of so-called "natural" foods. You might be surprised. And if you read the labels of some of the standard products on your grocery shelves, you'll find that some of them are processed without additives even though the manufacturers may not spend money boasting about the fact.

LEARN ABOUT LABELS: Foods are more accurately labeled these days than they used to be. In addition to a list of ingredients, many labels now provide information about the product's nutritional quality. Learn to pay attention to what the labels tell you, and you'll be able to get better nutrition for less cost.

You'll also need to learn what the labels *don't* tell you. As of 1976, for instance, nutrition labels list the Recommended Daily Allowances (RDA) for an "average" person (not necessarily you) of some, but *not* all, of the nutrients experts feel are needed for health. So if your pastry and orange-flavored drink add up to 100 percent of your RDA, you're still missing some of the essentials. Also, the nutritional quality is figured by a chemical analysis method that does not necessarily relate to a food's ability to provide nutrition for people.

SHOPPING TAKES SKILL: Being a consumer is not just a hobby; it's an important new role. Most people no longer grow their own food or make their own furniture. They buy it, and being a good buyer is as important as being a good farmer or carpenter. Schools, scouts and other organizations give courses in "consumerism." You might want to check them out. See page 135 for more ideas.

WHOM DO YOU TRUST?: You may also want to learn

a lot more about nutrition, by taking a course or by reading on your own. Learn all you can, but be sure of the sources of your information. Much of the material on food and nutrition is provided by people who have their own axes to grind or by corporations and organizations that have products to sell. Meat groups and dairy associations, for instance, can send you loads of useful material on nutritious cooking and eating, but they tend to stress the importance of meat or milk. So keep the source in mind when you're making use of the information.

LEARN TO COOK: For a minimum of artificial ingredients and the maximum of taste, cook it yourself. Chances are you already fix some of the family meals, at least on certain occasions. But if you do work in the kitchen, do you actually cook, or do you follow the directions on some package? Lots of people your age enjoy baking, but most of them probably think that means adding water and eggs to a mix. Cooking—real cooking, from "scratch"—is a creative experience. You'd be surprised how satisfying it can be to turn a few miscellaneous ingredients into a spectacular cake, casserole or soup.

When you start out, all you need do is follow the directions in a recipe. There are many good cookbooks, with simple, step-by-step instructions, no harder than those on the back of a package. See page 136 for a list. As you become more skillful, you can add your own touches, and what you create becomes an expression of yourself, rather than of some food technologist. While you're at it, learn to do it right. Learn how best to store and prepare food for maximum safety and food value.

GET TOGETHER: Once you've found that your cooking doesn't poison anyone, why not try potluck suppers? All your friends can gather at one house, each bringing something he or she has cooked. A party like that, or an after-school cooking club, can be more fun than munching potato chips all afternoon or evening.

And what about raising food? You can start a garden plot by yourself, of course, but it's more fun and less work if you can get a group together. You'll learn what it takes to produce food, you'll get to taste really fresh fruits and vegetables and you might even have some left over to sell. If you need help getting started (gardening takes more than dropping some seeds into the ground) your local agricultural extension service or 4-H Club can advise you.

FOLLOW YOUR CONSCIENCE: Once you begin thinking about your own food—about where it comes from and what it does for you—you may expand your thinking to a wider scale. If it bothers you to be fighting fat while many of your neighbors on this planet are fighting off starvation, you may want to eat more conscientiously. You can substitute grass-fed meats or nonmeat proteins for the grain-fed meats. You can make a practice of eating simple, unprocessed foods that don't waste as much of the earth's resources as the processed kinds.

YOU COUNT: Some people say that in a mass society, with mass production and mass marketing, the individual counts for little. But that isn't so. You count. You can change the way food is processed in this country by not casting your vote for foods that represent waste or empty calories. A quarter or a dollar won't make a difference, but if you join with others, you can be sure that manufacturers will get the message where they're most sensitive. Every worthwhile effort starts small and grows.

MINIMUM DAILY REQUIREMENTS
FOR THE AVERAGE TEEN-AGE DIET

Milk and milk products:	Four or more cups of milk or equivalent (1 cup milk = 1 cup yogurt, 1½ cups cottage cheese, 1-inch cube hard cheese or 2 cups ice cream)
Meat, fish, poultry:	Three 3-ounce servings or equivalent (1 serving = 2 eggs, 1 cup dried beans or 4 tablespoons peanut butter)
Green and/or yellow vegetables:	Two half-cup servings
Citrus fruits and other vitamin-C sources:	Two servings (1 serving = 6 ounces citrus juice, 8 ounces tomato juice, 1 orange, ½ grapefruit, 1 medium tomato or 2 cups lemonade)
Bread, cereals:	Four or more servings (1 serving = 1 slice bread, 1 ounce breakfast cereal or ½–¾ cup pasta)
Butter, oil, margarine:	2–4 tablespoons
Water:	32 ounces
Sweets and sugars:	None required

SOURCE: Deutsch, Ronald M., *The Family Guide to Better Food and Health* (Des Moines: Creative Library, 1971) from the Committee on Foods and Nutrition of the American Medical Association.

SURVIVING ON SNACKS

Nutritionists divide food into four main groups: *meat group* (meats, poultry, fish, eggs, with nuts and legumes as alternates); *milk group* (milk, cheese, ice cream, yogurt); *bread and cereal group* (whole-grain or enriched breads, cereals, pasta, rice and other grains); and *fruit and vegetable group* (citrus fruits, other fruits, leafy green vegetables, other vegetables including potatoes).

If you wish, you can meet your daily nutritional needs without ever sitting down to a "regular" meal, *if* you snack on the right foods. For instance:

... for "meat," pick up a pizza or a peanut-butter sandwich, nibble hard-boiled eggs, snack on nuts or a hamburger and try leftover cold chicken or roasts from the refrigerator;

... for "milk," eat ice-cream cones and other ice-cream snacks, try different flavors of yogurt, sip a milk shake, pick up another pizza, have cubes of cheese ready in the refrigerator, try a cheese sandwich or drink some milk;

... for "bread," make sure those sandwiches are made with whole-grain or enriched flours, buy muffins or a buttered roll if your day doesn't include a sandwich or pizza, nibble on crackers (there are some whole-wheat kinds) and popcorn (a good whole-grain);

... for "fruits and vegetables," buy orange, grapefruit or tomato juice instead of a soda; apples and raisins are good on-the-go snacks; oranges travel well and are a good source of vitamin C; keep raw vegetables cut up in plastic bags in the refrigerator (carrots, celery, cauliflower, broccoli, green beans, zucchini, cucumbers and radishes all keep well); dip the vegetables in mayonnaise or salad dressing to get some of your fat allowance; spinach, head lettuce and cabbage are good when eaten in chunks; but don't count potato chips or french fries as a "vegetable," as potatoes lose much of their food value during standard processing techniques;

... you'll have no trouble meeting your requirement for fats and oils, especially if you spread your sandwiches with butter or margarine;

... drink water from a fountain or from the tap; it's free with meals in restaurants, and it's a lot better for you than soda pop.

GETTING THE FACTS ON
PROTEINS, CARBOHYDRATES
AND FATS

PROTEINS

Proteins are made of amino acids. The body needs more than 20 different amino acids, but it can manufacture all but eight of them. These eight are essential to your diet. It is also important that they be eaten together, rather than at separate meals. Amino acids are available in a wide variety of foods, not just in so-called "protein foods."

Most foods containing protein contain *all* the essential amino acids (but there are a few exceptions). A "high-quality" protein is one that contains those eight essential amino acids in the correct proportions for use by humans. A "low-quality" protein is low in one or more of the essential amino acids and therefore it cannot be used as efficiently by the human body.

If you are aged 11 to 14, you need 1 gram of protein for each kilogram of your body's weight. If you are aged 15 to 18, multiply the number of kilograms you weigh by .89. (A kilogram is approximately 2.2 pounds.) The result will equal the number of grams of protein you need each day. These figures are averages—if you eat mainly high-quality proteins, you may need slightly less; if you eat mainly low-quality proteins, you may need slightly more. Depending on your age and weight, you probably need about 45 grams of protein a day.

"Straight proteins" are foods that provide complete, high-quality protein all by themselves. Here are some examples:

food/serving	grams of protein
whole milk, 1 cup	9
egg, 1 whole	6
meat, fish or poultry, 3 oz.	15–25
uncreamed cottage cheese, 2 oz.	10
ice cream, ½ cup	3

So, if you drank a quart of milk and ate two ounces of cottage cheese, you would more than meet your daily protein requirement.

"Complementary proteins" are two proteins which, when eaten together, provide a better quality protein than either one individually. The essential amino acids low in one food are supplied by the other, and vice-versa. But calculating the useable protein in complementary foods is very complex and still controversial.

food/serving	grams of protein
cheese pizza	about 10 per slice
cereal with milk	about 8.5 per cup
rice and beans	about 10 per serving

Complementary protein dishes usually cost less, are lower in calories and lower in fat than "straight protein" dishes. For more information on protein needs and sources, see the books listed on pages 130–132.

CARBOHYDRATES

Carbohydrates are simple combinations of carbon, hydrogen and oxygen atoms. They are easily broken down by the body and therefore are useful for energy as well as other purposes. Some carbohydrates that cannot be digested provide necessary "roughage."

"Low-carbohydrate" diets are often in vogue, but they are pointless because carbohydrates have the same calorie count as protein—about four calories per gram. Low-carbohydrate diets can also be dangerous because they may upset the system's vital balance.

Carbohydrates should make up about 40 percent of the adolescent diet, with 100 grams per day as the bare minimum. Carbohydrates are easy to obtain because they abound in practically every food but meats, eggs and some cheeses. The trick is to get other nutrients along with the carbohydrates. Fruits, vegetables, grain products and milk tend to be high in carbohydrates and are also essential to the diet. Candy, sugar, soda and most commercial snack foods provide carbohydrates with almost no other nutrients. That is why they are called "empty calories."

FATS

Fats are made up of "fatty acids." Fatty acids are chains of carbon, hydrogen and fewer oxygen atoms. The arrangement of the fatty acids determines whether the fat is liquid, like cooking oil, or solid, like shortening. The particular combination of fatty acids gives a fat its special taste: butter tastes different from lard because it contains a different group of fatty acids.

A fat is saturated, unsaturated or polyunsaturated, depending upon the form of its fatty-acid chains. In a saturated fat the carbon atoms are linked to as many hydrogen atoms as they can hold; it is "saturated" with hydrogen.

An unsaturated fat has space left in the chain for hydrogen atoms. A polyunsaturated fat has many spaces left empty.

The body uses fats for stored energy, for warmth and for padding. Fats are also essential in the functioning of other nutrients. "Fat-soluable" vitamins A, D, E and K, for instance, are not effective without fat.

Saturated fats can act to raise the level of cholesterol in the bloodstream. Cholesterol is a substance somewhat (but not exactly) like a fat. Cholesterol is found in egg yolks and organ meats (liver, kidneys, etc.) but it is also produced by the body and used in the construction of cell walls. Excess cholesterol in the bloodstream can be deposited along the walls of the blood vessels. As layers of cholesterol build up, the blood has less and less room to flow. Heart disease, stroke and other disorders can be the result. Unsaturated fats do not increase the body's cholesterol level and polyunsaturated fats can lower the cholesterol count.

Fats in the diet come from animal sources: in butter, milk, eggs and the skins and flesh of meat, poultry and fish; and from vegetable sources: seeds and nuts and the oils made from them. Saturated fats predominate in meats and dairy products. Olive oil and peanut oil are the most common unsaturated fats. Polyunsaturated fats come in the form of corn oil, soybean oil, safflower oil, cottonseed oil and margarine made from those oils.

At nine calories per gram, fats contain more than twice the food energy of proteins or carbohydrates, and fats are more easily stored by the body. So, overintake of fats can lead to obesity and all its complications. Some research suggests that a diet heavy in fats may be linked to a variety of other disorders, including some types of cancer. A diet heavy in saturated fats, as the American diet tends to be, can cause heart and artery disease and other cholesterol-related problems.

Teen-agers should get approximately 40 percent of their calories in the form of fats. And adolescence is not too early to be conscious of eating the right kinds of fat. Boys, especially, can start storing cholesterol from a young age, and the problem only increases as they grow older. Women usually do not seem to have a problem with cholesterol until after menopause, but individual patterns vary.

Teen-agers without a diagnosed medical problem should *not* avoid meats, eggs and dairy products, because important vitamins and minerals accompany the saturated fats and cholesterol. But teen-agers should also take in some of their fats in unsaturated and polyunsaturated forms as well.

NUTRITION CHART

NUTRIENTS	AMOUNT NEEDED				SOURCES IN THE FOOD SUPPLY	USES IN THE BODY
	BOYS 11-14	BOYS 15-18	GIRLS 11-14	GIRLS 15-18		
Calories	2800	3000	2400	2100	All foods contain calories. Adolescents should take in about 20% of their calories as protein, 40% as carbohydrates and 40% as fats.	Calories measure the energy value of food. The amount of energy required depends upon the energy used for growth, maintenance and activity.
Protein	44gm	54gm	44gm	48gm	Meats, fish, poultry, eggs, milk, whole grains, beans, some other vegetables and combinations of "incomplete" proteins.	Proteins build cells in almost every solid and fluid part of the body; they form regulatory enzymes and disease-fighting antibodies.
Carbohydrates	Daily allowance not established, but should constitute 40% of your calorie intake				Sugars and sweetened foods, cereals and grains, baked goods, fruits, vegetables, milk.	Carbohydrates are the principal source of energy for all the body's functions. They also provide material for cell walls and contribute to regulatory processes.
Fats	Daily allowance not established, but should constitute 40% of your calorie intake				Meats, fish, poultry, egg yolk, whole milk, cheese, butter, margarine, oils, nuts.	Fats are stored for energy, warmth and padding. Fats carry "fat-soluble" vitamins and interact with other nutrients for proper functioning.

					Drinking water.	Forms body fluids; regulates temperature; removes wastes; carries nutrients; provides some minerals.
Water		1½-2 quarts fluid				
Fat-Soluble Vitamins						
Vitamin A	5000IU	5000IU	4000IU	4000IU	Liver, fish-liver oils, butter, whole milk and whole-milk cheeses, fortified margarine and skim milk, squash, carrots, dark-green leafy vegetables.	Helps normal formation of bones and teeth; skin and mucous membrane health; good night vision and healthy eyes.
Vitamin D	400IU	400IU	400IU	400IU	Sunlight, fortified milk and some egg yolks, fish and liver.	Works with calcium and phosphorus to build bones and teeth; helps body make use of protein.
Vitamin E	12IU	12IU	12IU	12IU	Seed and soybean oils, wheat germ, some nuts, leafy green vegetables, liver, margarine.	Protects Vitamin A and fatty acids in the body.
Vitamin K	(Daily allowance not established)				Many green vegetables, egg yolk and pork liver.	Helps the blood to clot.

NUTRITION CHART

| NUTRIENTS | AMOUNT NEEDED | | | | SOURCES IN THE FOOD SUPPLY | USES IN THE BODY |
	BOYS 11-14	BOYS 15-18	GIRLS 11-14	GIRLS 15-18		
Water-Soluble Vitamins						
Vitamin C	45mg	45mg	45mg	45mg	Citrus fruits and juices, tomatoes and juice, melons and other fruits, many green vegetables, potatoes, and foods enriched with Vitamin C.	Helps form connective tissue and blood hemoglobin; helps enzymes function; helps body make use of iron and perhaps protein and carbohydrates. Promotes healing of wounds and helps ward off infection.
Folic Acid	400μ	400μ	400μ	400μ	Liver, dried beans, nuts, whole-grain breads and cereals, dark green vegetables.	A "B-type" vitamin. Helps cells build and function; helps enzymes function; helps formation of red blood cells.
Niacin	18mg	20mg	16mg	12mg	Poultry, fish, organ meats, wheat germ, whole-grain bread; enriched bread, beans, nuts and seeds.	A "B-type" vitamin. Helps body produce energy and use fats; vital for healthy tissues.
Riboflavin (Vitamin B_2)	1.5mg	1.8mg	1.3mg	1.4mg	Milk, whey, cheese, eggs, butter, liver, kidney, heart, other meats, beans, leafy greens, enriched bread.	Helps body make use of proteins, fats and carbohydrates.

					Food Sources	Function
Thiamin (Vitamin B_1)	1.4mg	1.5mg	1.2mg	1.1mg	Meats, fish, poultry, liver, whole grains, wheat germ, seeds, nuts, some leafy vegetables.	Helps body make use of carbohydrates; promotes good appetite, digestion and healthy nerves.
Vitamin B_6	1.6mg	2mg	1.6mg	2mg	Wheat germ, whole grains, seeds, some nuts and beans, meats and organ meats, potatoes and some green vegetables.	Helps body make use of proteins and fats, and to form niacin.
Vitamin B_{12}	3mg	3mg	3mg	3mg	Meats, fish, poultry, eggs, milk and milk products.	Needed for internal structure of cells; helps body form an amino acid; used in formation of red blood cells.
Biotin	(Daily allowance not established)				Organ meats, egg yolk, milk, nuts and many other foods.	Helps body make use of proteins, fats and carbohydrates, among other functions.
Pantothenic Acid	(Daily allowance not established)				Found in most foods, especially organ meats, wheat germ and whole grains.	Helps body make use of proteins, fats and carbohydrates, among other functions.
Minerals						
Calcium	1200mg	1200mg	1200mg	1200mg	Milk, cheese, dark-green leafy vegetables.	Needed for strong bones and teeth; for proper function of muscles, including the heart; for blood clotting; helps enzymes function.

NUTRITION CHART

NUTRIENTS	AMOUNT NEEDED				SOURCES IN THE FOOD SUPPLY	USES IN THE BODY
	BOYS 11-14	BOYS 15-18	GIRLS 11-14	GIRLS 15-18		
Magnesium	350mg	400mg	300mg	300mg	Whole grains, nuts, beans, milk and some vegetables.	Helps body make use of carbohydrates; helps regulate muscles, nerves and blood.
Phosphorus	1200mg	1200mg	1200mg	1200mg	Milk, eggs, cheese, organ meats, meat, fish, whole grains, some peas and beans.	Helps body make use of fats and carbohydrates; needed for strong bones and teeth; for muscle function and cell wall formation.
Chlorine	(Daily allowance not established)				Salt.	Helps form necessary acids and maintain acid-base balance.
Potassium	(Daily allowance not established)				Many foods, especially bananas, dates, melons, dark-green vegetables and meats.	Works with sodium to maintain body's fluid balance, nerve and muscle regulation; helps body make use of carbohydrates and fats.
Sodium	(Daily allowance not established)				Salt and salted foods, milk, cheese, eggs, meat, some vegetables.	Helps maintain body's fluid balance, regulates muscles and nerves.
Sulfur	(Daily allowance not established)				Meat, milk, cheese, peas, beans and nuts.	Makes up some amino acids and is part of thiamin and biotin.

"Trace" Minerals						
Iodine	130μ	150μ	115μ	115μ	Seafood, plants and animals grown near the seacoast, iodized salt.	Vital to hormones produced by the thyroid gland for regulation of growth and basic body functions.
Iron	18mg	18mg	18mg	18mg	Liver and other organ meats, meats, shellfish, prunes, raisins and some other fruits, beans and peas, whole grains, nuts, green leafy vegetables.	Part of every cell; essential to the blood's ability to carry oxygen throughout the body.
Zinc	15mg	15mg	15mg	15mg	Fish and seafood, meats and poultry, wheat germ and whole grains, beans and nuts.	Makes up enzymes needed for the body to use proteins and carbohydrates.
Chromium	(Daily allowance not established)				Whole grains, meats.	Helps the body make use of fats and carbohydrates.
Copper	(Daily allowance not established)				In most foods except milk and dairy products.	Helps form blood hemoglobin; helps the body use carbohydrates.
Fluorine	(Daily allowance not established)				Water, fluoridated naturally or artificially; fish.	Needed for healthy teeth.

NUTRITION CHART

NUTRIENTS	AMOUNT NEEDED				SOURCES IN THE FOOD SUPPLY	USES IN THE BODY
	BOYS 11-14	BOYS 15-18	GIRLS 11-14	GIRLS 15-18		
Manganese	(Daily allowance not established)				Many foods, especially whole grains, beans, meats and dark leafy vegetables.	Helps form and activate many enzymes; helps body make use of fats and carbohydrates.
Fiber	(Daily allowance not established)				Vegetables, fruits, whole grains, beans, nuts.	Helps keep bowels active and the digestive system efficient.

SOURCES:

"Recommended Dietary Allowances" (Food and Nutrition Board, National Academy of Sciences, 1974).

Mayer, Jean, *A Diet for Living* (New York: McKay, 1975).

Robinson, Corinne H., *Fundamentals of Normal Nutrition* (New York: Macmillan, 1972).

White, Philip L., and Selvey, Nancy, *Let's Talk About Food* (Chicago: Follett, 1975).

ADDITIVES CHART

NAME	PURPOSE	IS IT SAFE?
Acetic Acid	To preserve, flavor and add tartness to foods.	Yes.
Adipic Acid	To flavor soft drinks and dessert and drink powders; to preserve oils.	Yes.
Alginate	Seaweed extract used to thicken and give smooth consistency to ice cream, candy, yogurt, frosting, whipped cream and other foods.	Yes.
Amylases	Natural enzymes used in breadmaking, brewing and other processes.	Yes—nutritious, too.
Ascorbic Acid (Vitamin C)	To fortify foods; to preserve freshness in foods containing fats; to treat bread dough.	Yes—except that overintake of Vitamin C may have bad side effects.
Brominated Vegetable Oil (BVO)	To hold flavoring agents in soft drinks.	No—and it does not have to be listed on the label.
Butylated Hydroxy-anisole (BHA) Butylated Hydroxy-toluene (BHT)	To increase shelf life of many products, including vegetable oils, candy, potato chips, cereals and mixes.	The FDA considers them safe, but many scientists say they've been improperly tested and offer more risks than benefits, especially as they accumulate in the body over time.

Caffeine	To jazz up flavor of cola-type soft drinks; occurs naturally in cocoa, chocolate and coffee.	Anything more than a small amount can produce a variety of harmful effects.
Calcium and Sodium Proprionate	To preserve freshness in baked goods.	Yes.
Carotene	Used to color and/or fortify foods like margarine, milk, mixes and other foods.	Yes—the body converts this yellow pigment to Vitamin A. But overintake of Vitamin A can be harmful.
Carrageenan	Seaweed extract used to improve texture of milk products and thicken jelly, syrup and other foods, including infant formulas.	Yes, in general, but it may be dangerous for infants.
Casein	Milk protein that improves the texture and/or whitens frozen desserts and other products.	Yes—nutritious, too.
Cellulose Gum and CMC	Used to improve texture of a variety of foods; derivatives are used as fillers.	Yes.
Chewing Gum Bases	A variety of natural and/or synthetic substances used to make chewing gum chewable.	Perhaps not; they have not been adequately tested.
Citric Acid	Flavors and preserves the freshness of a wide variety of foods.	Yes.

ADDITIVES CHART

NAME	PURPOSE	IS IT SAFE?
Coloring Agents	Virtually all types of food that are processed in any way contain some form of added color. Even foods that don't look red, for example, may have been perked up with red coloring. Coloring agents may be dyes derived from coal tar, synthetic chemicals or natural products such as paprika, carrots or beets. Coloring agents contribute nothing to the nutritive value of food.	Colors used in foods must be officially proven safe, or "certified." This does not mean that every dose of a given color *is* safe, and the safety tests have been widely criticized. Coal-tar dyes are especially suspect. Consumers have no way of knowing what agents have been used in a food that calls itself "artificially colored," and many types of food do not even have to carry that information on the label. To be as safe as possible from dangerous dyes, one would have to avoid all "artificially colored" foods unless the label specified a safe color, such as "Caramel Coloring Added."
Dextrin	A starch. Various starches are used to thicken foods, to carry flavors and to maintain texture.	Dextrin and other natural starches are safe and nutritious. Some types of "modified starches," often found in frozen foods or pie fillings, may be hazardous.
EDTA	This acid is used to trap bits of metal scraped off machinery during processing, preserve freshness and prevent discoloration in a variety of foods and drinks.	Yes.

Additive	Use	Safe?
Flavorings	Artificial flavorings include a wide variety of chemicals used alone or in combination to create or enhance the taste of processed foods.	Many are not widely considered safe; many have not been tested. A label need only state "artificial flavoring," without indicating what chemicals were used.
Fumaric Acid	Adds tartness to dry products.	Yes.
Glycerin, Glycerol	Added to keep candy, baked goods and other foods moist.	Yes.
Guar Gum	Plant extract used to thicken many foods and treat bread dough.	Yes.
Hydrolized Vegetable Protein (HVP)	Plant protein broken down chemically into amino acids.	Yes.
Lactic Acid	Preserves and/or adds flavor to a variety of foods.	Generally yes, though perhaps not for infants.
Lecithin	Used to preserve freshness of fats in foods, and to improve texture of a variety of products.	Yes—nutritious, too.
Malic Acid	Adds tartness and flavor to a variety of foods.	Natural malic acid is safe; synthetic malic acid may not be safe for babies.
Mono- and Di-glycerides	Used to preserve freshness and improve texture of a wide variety of foods, including margarine, bread and peanut butter.	Yes, but they may replace more nourishing ingredients, and some of their derivatives may not have been well tested.

ADDITIVES CHART

NAME	PURPOSE	IS IT SAFE?
Monosodium Glutamate (MSG)	Used to enhance the flavor of a variety of foods.	Generally yes, but large amounts may produce side effects, and MSG may be harmful to unborn and newborn babies.
Polysorbates	"Emulsifiers" that disperse flavors in foods and keep some foods fresh.	Probably.
Propyl Gallate	Used to preserve freshness somewhat.	FDA considers it safe, but other scientists say it has not been well tested and may be harmful.
Sodium Benzoate	Used to preserve freshness in acid foods.	Yes, though links to birth defects may not have been well enough tested.
Sodium Nitrate, Sodium Nitrite	Used to preserve and color "cured" meats like ham, hot dogs and bologna, and to protect them from botulism.	No. While they are useful and safe in small quantities, they can be dangerous in large amounts and they combine with other substances to form cancer-causing agents in laboratory animals. The amount needed to protect meat from botulism is only a small fraction of the amount usually added by food processors.

Sugar and Sweeteners	A variety of natural and synthetic substances used to sweeten and perk up the flavor of many foods.	Corn syrup—yes; dextrose—yes; glucose—yes; fructose—yes; invert sugar—yes; lactose—yes; mannitol—yes; saccharine—probably; sucrose—yes. All these sugars (except saccharine) contribute to cavities and to obesity which leads to many ills. Otherwise, these sugars are "safe."
Tannin	Chemical made from bark, used for flavor and other purposes in many foods; occurs naturally in coffee, tea and cocoa.	FDA considers it safe, but some scientists suspect it may contribute to cancer.
Texturized Vegetable Protein (TVP)	Protein from plants, usually soybeans, that is broken down and rearranged in other forms to resemble a variety of foods.	TVP itself is safe and nutritious; flavorings and other ingredients added to make it imitate other foods may not be.
Whey	Milk byproduct used as filler, texturizer and enriching additive in many foods.	Yes—nutritious, too.

In addition to this partial list of additives are substances like pesticides, growth hormones and antibiotics which enter the food supply before the processing stage. Residues of these chemicals may remain in the food, and some may be harmful.

SOURCES:

Jacobson, Michael F., *Eater's Digest* (New York: Anchor Books, 1972).

Potter, Norman N., *Food Science* (Westport, Conn.: AVI, 1973).

U.S. Food and Drug Administration. Various publications.

White, Philip L., and Selvey, Nancy, *Let's Talk About Food* (Publishing Sciences Group, 1974).

WHERE TO FIND OUT MORE

NUTRITION

READ:

American Dietetic Association, *Food Facts Talk Back.*
Available for 75¢ from the American Dietetic Association, 430 N. Michigan Ave., Chicago, Ill. 60611.
> A short but thorough pamphlet on nutrition. The Association is a good source for a variety of materials on nutrition and diet.

Deutsch, Ronald M., *The Family Guide to Better Food and Better Health* (New York: Bantam Books, 1973).
> A complete, readable survey of food, dieting and nutrition.

Goodhart, R. S., *The Teen-Ager's Guide to Diet and Health* (Englewood Cliffs, N.J.: Prentice-Hall, 1964).
> A useful introduction.

Jacobson, Michael F., *Nutrition Scoreboard* (New York: Avon Books, 1975).
> A practical guide to getting good nutrition from available foods, plus other information on the American way of eating.

Lappé, Frances Moore, *Diet for a Small Planet* (New York: Ballantine Books, 1975).
> Explains the need for getting protein from non-meat sources, and outlines ways to do it.

Leverton, Ruth M., *Food Becomes You* (Ames, Ia: Iowa State University Press, 1965).
> Easy-to-read introduction to nutrition.

Mayer, Jean, *A Diet for Living* (New York: David McKay, 1975).
    Nutritional information for all ages, in question-and-answer form.

————, *Protein—How Much Is Enough?* Available for 50¢ and a stamped, self-addressed envelope from Newspaperbooks, 800 Third Ave., New York, N.Y. 10022.
    A small pamphlet explaining uses and multiple sources of protein.

McWilliams, Margaret, *Nutrition for the Growing Years* (New York: John Wiley, 1967).
    A textbook focusing on food needs from infancy through adolescence.

Salmon, M. S., *Food Facts for Teen-Agers* (Springfield, Ill.: Chas. C. Thomas, 1965).
    A simply written summary of nutrition.

U.S. Department of Agriculture, *Composition of Foods*. Available for $2.35 from the Superintendent of Documents, Government Printing Office, Washington, D.C. 20402.
    Complete listing of the nutrients in practically every food.

————, *Nutrition: Food at Work for You*. Available for 20¢ from the Supt. of Documents, GPO.
    A short, handy guide to nutrition and food preparation and storage.

U.S. Department of Health, Education and Welfare, *Facts About Nutrition*. Available for 35¢ from Supt. of Documents, GPO.
    Nutritional summary and diet suggestions.

White, Philip L., and Selvey, Nancy, *Let's Talk About Food* (Chicago: Follett, 1974).
    Readable information about food, diet and food processing from the American Medical Association.

Wilson, Eva D.; Fisher, Katherine H.; and Fuqua, Mary
E., *Principles of Nutrition* (New York: John Wiley,
1975).
A textbook, thorough and up-to-date.

Zim, Herbert, *Your Food and You* (New York: William
Morrow, 1957).
A *very* simple introduction to nutrition.

CONTACT:

Dial-a-Dietician: check your phone book to see if your
local government has a number you can dial for nutrition information.

Your state or local health department or the USDA cooperative extension service probably provides nutritional
information or courses. Check it out.

The Information Divisions of the Food and Nutrition
Service and the Agricultural Research Service of the U.S.
Department of Agriculture (Washington, D.C. 20250)
provide a variety of material on food and nutrition, much
of it free. Write them.

The Consumer Information Center, Public Documents
Distribution Center, Pueblo, Colo. 81009, is a government
agency that will put you on the mailing list for catalogs
of consumer information pamphlets, which include nutritional material, if you write and ask.

DIETING

READ:

Berland, Theodore, and the Editors of *Consumer Guide*,
Rating the Diets (Skokie, Ill.: Publications International,
1974).
A brief discussion of the causes of overweight and a
close look at all the ways, good and bad, of getting
rid of it.

Gilbert, Sara, *Fat Free* (New York: Macmillan, 1975). The author's book for teen-agers about fat, feelings about fat and ways to get rid of it or stop worrying about it.

Gregg, Walter H., *A Boy and His Physique.* Available from the National Dairy Council, 111 North Canal Street, Chicago, Ill. 60606.
A pamphlet on weight control, nutrition and "body-building." Brief but sound, with only moderate over-emphasis on dairy products.

Leverton, Ruth M., *A Girl and Her Figure.* Available from the National Dairy Council (see above).
A good, short pamphlet on dieting and exercise, with stress on the need for milk.

Mayer, Jean, *Overweight* (Englewood Cliffs, N.J.: Prentice-Hall, 1968).
A book on the causes and cures of obesity, intended for adults, with a chapter on adolescent fat.

U.S. Department of Agriculture, *Food and Your Weight.* Available for 50¢ from the Superintendent of Documents, Government Printing Office, Washington, D.C. 20402.
A good handbook on dieting and calories, with emphasis on adults.

FOOD PROCESSING AND ADDITIVES

READ:

Consumer Reports (Box 1000, Orangeburg, N.Y. 10962) Monthly magazine and year-end annual book available on newsstands, in libraries and by subscription.
Reports of Consumers' Union include many test results on foods and additives.

Hightower, Jim, *Eat Your Heart Out* (New York: Crown, 1975).
A detailed examination of the food industry by a critic of the system.

Jacobson, Michael F., *Eater's Digest* (New York: Anchor Books, 1972).
A close analysis of many of the major food additives, including pro's and con's about their use, along with a brief summary of the food-processing system.

Lerza, Catherine, and Jacobson, Michael, eds., *Food for People, Not Profit* (New York: Ballantine Books, 1975).
A collection of articles on the food industry, additives and hunger by writers generally critical of the system. Includes suggestions on ways to take action toward solutions.

Margolius, Sidney, *The Great American Food Hoax* (New York: Walker, 1971).
A generally critical, but reasonable, look at the pitfalls in the American way of eating, with ideas on how to avoid them.

Verrett, Jacqueline, and Carper, Jean, *Eating May be Hazardous to Your Health* (New York: Simon & Schuster, 1974).
A scary, but apparently accurate, book by a former researcher for FDA, presenting the "case against food additives."

Winter, Ruth, *Consumer's Dictionary of Food Additives* (New York: Crown, 1972).
A listing of food additives, their functions and possible dangers.

CONTACT:

For more information, or for help in taking action on food-processing issues, write these organizations that are fighting the system:

Agribusiness Accountability Project
1000 Wisconsin Avenue, NW
Washington, D.C. 20007

Center for Science in the Public Interest
1779 Church Street, NW
Washington, D.C. 20036

BUYING

READ:

Consumer Reports (See above)
Magazine offers comparisons of cost and quality in articles on food.

Gay, Kathlyn, *Be a Smart Shopper* (New York: Julian Messner, 1974).
An introduction to wise buying for young readers.

Goldberg, Nikki and David, *The Supermarket Handbook* (New York: Harper & Row, 1973).
A good guide to buying the most nutrition, with the least adulteration, conveniently.

Saunders, Rubie, *Smart Shopping and Consumerism* (New York: Franklin Watts, 1973).
An easy-to-read summary of buying tips.

U.S. Department of Agriculture, *Your Money's Worth in Foods*. Available for 50¢ from the Superintendent of Documents, Government Printing Office, Washington, D.C. 20402.
This and other USDA publications offer practical ideas for buying and caring for food.

CONTACT:

Your local school, college, health department, Scouts, YWCA, 4-H Club, agricultural extensions service or other organizations probably have courses in how to be a wise consumer. Check them out.

If for any reason you are unsatisfied with any food you buy or eat, by all means, complain! Write to:

The manufacturer, at the address on the label.

Your local Consumer Affairs Office, listed in the phone book.

U.S. Office of Consumer Affairs
Washington, D.C. 20201

Food and Drug Administration
5600 Fishers Lane
Rockville, Md. 20852
    (for complaints about labeling or hazards)

Federal Trade Commission
Washington, D.C. 20580
    (for complaints about advertising or marketing)

COOKING

READ:

Anderson, Jean, and Hanna, Elaine, *The Doubleday Cookbook* (New York: Doubleday, 1975).
    Without question the best basic cookbook available for cooks at any level of experience. Includes nutritional information and calorie counts along with many other food facts.

Ewald, Ellen Buchman, *Recipes for a Small Planet* (New York: Ballantine, 1973).
    "Complementary protein" recipes, like those in *Diet for a Small Planet*, but more of them.

The Fanny Farmer Cookbook (New York: Bantam Books, 1972).
    The classic American cookbook, revised and updated, in paperback.

Katz, Martha Ellen, *The Complete Book of High-Protein Baking* (New York: Ballantine, 1975).
How to make "sweets" and "starches" into protein foods.

Rombauer, Irma S., and Becker, Marion Rombauer, *The Joy of Cooking* (New York: New American Library, 1975).
Another all-inclusive basic cookbook, in paperback.

U.S. Department of Agriculture, *Family Fare.* Available for $1.00 from Superintendent of Documents, Government Printing Office, Washington, D.C. 20402.
A short collection of recipes and food information.

Note:
The above listing includes only a few of the thousands of basic and specialized cookbooks available. You might enjoy browsing through the cookbook section of your library or bookstore for others.

FOOD AND CULTURE

READ:

Berry, Erick, *Eating and Cooking Around the World— Fingers Before Forks* (New York: John Day, 1963).
A simply written book about food customs of different societies.

Johnson, Lois S., *What We Eat* (Chicago: Rand-McNally, 1969).
An easy-to-read history of many common foods, and a look at future diets.

Tannahill, Reay, *Food in History* (New York: Stein and Day, 1973).
A lengthy but fascinating account of the central role food has played in culture since prehistoric times.

HUNGER AND FOOD SHORTAGES

READ:

Kotz, Nick, *Let Them Eat Promises* (Englewood Cliffs, N.J.: Prentice-Hall, 1969).
An interesting and disturbing account, intended for adults, of "the politics of hunger in America."

Pringle, Laurence, *Our Hungry Earth* (New York: Macmillan, 1976).
A simply and carefully written discussion of the world food shortage.

Vicker, Ray, *This Hungry World* (New York: Scribner, 1975).
A readable, detailed account, intended for adults, of present and potential starvation.

Note:
In addition to books like the above devoted entirely to the food crisis, most current books on food contain sections on the topic. See, for instance, Lerza and Jacobson, or Lappé.

"CONSCIENTIOUS EATING"

READ:

Deutsch, Ronald M., *Nuts Among the Berries* (New York: Ballantine, 1962).
A humorous but accurate discussion of food fads, to read before taking any "health-food" plunge.

Fenter, Barbara and D. X., *Natural Foods* (New York: Franklin Watts, 1974).
An unusually sensible and reasonable introduction to a diet that avoids over-refined and over-adulterated foods; includes a section debunking food myths.

Hunter, Beatrice Trum, *The Natural Foods Primer* (New York: Simon & Schuster, 1972).
Another sanely written, practical guide to eating simply and safely.

Lappé, Frances Moore, *Diet for a Small Planet.*
See page 130.

Margolius, Sidney, *Health Foods: Facts and Fakes* (New York: Walker, 1973).
Factual presentation of the sense and nonsense surrounding health foods. Excerpts from the book are available as a pamphlet under the same title for 35¢ from Public Affairs Pamphlets, 381 Park Ave. South, New York, N.Y. 10016.

CONTACT:

If you want advice on improving the snacks available in your school, write:

Jean Farmer
Cedarwood Press
1115 E. Wylie St.
Bloomington, Ind. 47401
(enclose a stamped, self-addressed envelope)

If you are interested in ways to effectively "share" your food with the hungry, contact:

CARE, Inc.
660 First Ave.
New York, N.Y. 10016

International Red Cross
150 Amsterdam Ave.
New York, N.Y. 10023

International Rescue Committee
386 Park Ave. South
New York, N.Y. 10016

U.S. Committee for UNICEF
331 East 38th Street
New York, N.Y. 10016

Many national youth groups and religious organizations have hunger-fighting projects. Check them out.

INDEX